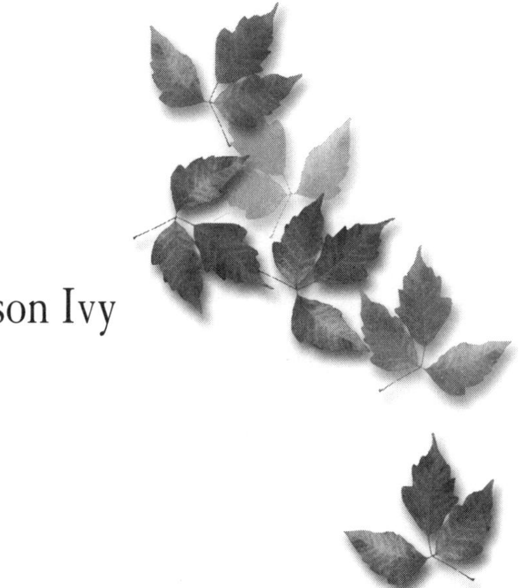

Attacked by Poison Ivy

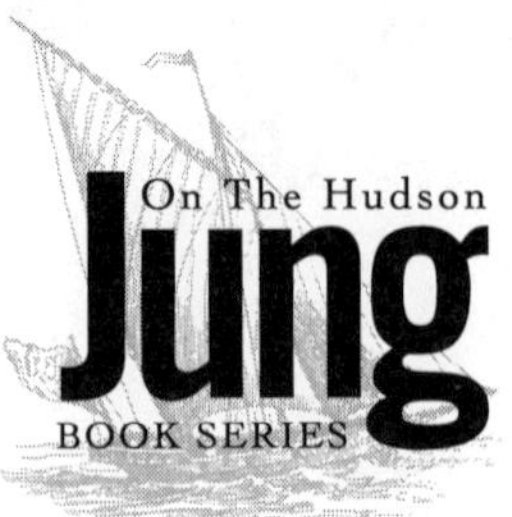

The Jung on the Hudson Book Series was instituted by the New York Center for Jungian Studies in 1997. This ongoing series is designed to present books that will be of interest to individuals of all fields, as well as mental health professionals, who are interested in exploring the relevance of the psychology and ideas of C. G. Jung to their personal lives and professional activities.

For more information about this series and the New York Center for Jungian Studies contact: Aryeh Maidenbaum, Ph.D., New York Center for Jungian Studies, 41 Park Avenue, Suite 1D, New York, NY 10016, telephone (212) 689-8238, fax (212) 889-7634.

For more information about becoming part of this series contact: Nicolas-Hays, P. O. Box 2039, York Beach, ME 03910-2039.

ATTACKED *by* POISON IVY

A Psychological Understanding

ANN BELFORD ULANOV

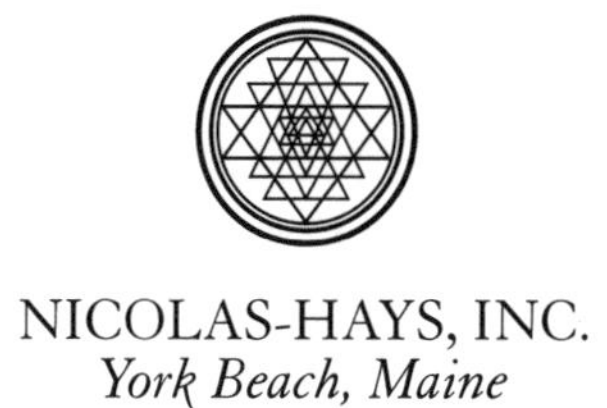

NICOLAS-HAYS, INC.
York Beach, Maine

First published in 2001 by
Nicolas-Hays, Inc.
Box 2039
York Beach, ME 03910

Distributed to the trade by
Red Wheel/Weiser, LLC
368 Congress Street
Boston, MA 02210

Library of Congress Cataloging-in-Publication Data
Ulanov, Ann Belford.
Attacked by poison ivy : a psychological understanding / Ann Belford Ulanov.
p. cm. "A Jung on the Hudson Book"
Includes bibliographical references and index.
ISBN 0-89254-058-3 (pbk. : alk. paper)
1. Poison ivy—Psychosomatic aspects. 2. Jungian psychology. I. Title
RA1242.R4 U56 2001
615.9'52377—dc21 2001032606

TCP
Cover and text design by Kathryn Sky-Peck
Typeset in 11.5/18 Granjon

Printed in Canada

08 07 06 05 04 03 02 01
8 7 6 5 4 3 2 1

The paper used in this publication meets the minimum requirements of the American National Standard for Information Sciences—Permanence of Paper for Printed Library Materials Z39.48-1992 (R1997).

To Barry

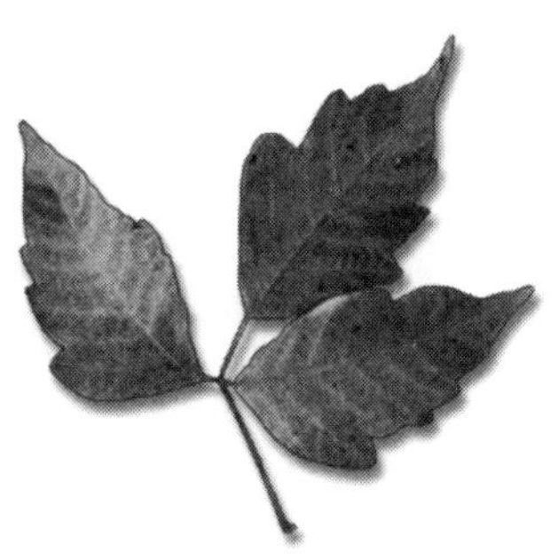

CONTENTS

ACKNOWLEDGMENTS

I warmly acknowledge the help of Aryeh Maidenbaum in locating this book with Betty Lundsted of Nicolas-Hays, Inc. My warmest thanks to Betty Lundsted for her editorial skills, always rendered with tact, courtesy, and enthusiasm for the work. My thanks as well to other members of the Ivy League; we have shared this suffering.

FOREWORD

By Stephen Larsen

On the island of Sri Lanka, adjacent to Southern India, some twenty-five years ago, my wife Robin and I studied the masked "devil dancers" whose presence clearly speaks of a religion older than the Buddhism manifested in the giant stupas and meditating Buddhas everywhere. The ceremonies are an "animistic" leftover, say the anthropologists, for in mandalic drawings in the sand, dance the fierce, grinning, and tusked masks of the spirits of many illnesses: syphilis, typhoid, cholera, even schizophrenia, in rituals that include both manifestation and containment, dramatization and *gnosis* of the illness. The rituals, later integrated into Buddhism, imply that illnesses contain a spiritual essence that can be recognized and known.[1]

This is a remarkable revelation, this transformation of illness into image, pathology into mask. But there is a myth which explains it: In ancient times the sickness-demons beset Earth and killed many people everywhere. People prayed to the Great

Buddha to save them from this affliction, but the chief of the sickness-demons, *Maha Kola Sanniya Yakṣaya*, appeared before the World-Savior and told him that there were two sides to the story. If he and his sickness-demons desisted entirely, human beings would become complacent and self-satisfied. It was only when human beings were afflicted with illness, the crafty demon asserted, that they became religious, rolling their eyes heavenward, begging for mercy, and vowing to mend their ways. The Buddha meditated long and hard, finally decreeing that the demons should still have the right to make mankind ill, but not to kill wantonly; and if the people made masks of the demons and danced in these sacred mandalic enclosures, their rituals would also have the efficacy to heal the illnesses the demons had brought.

In this mythology, an ancient insight into the "other side of illness" is taught. The myth is the primordial explanation of the ever-renewed dramatic ritual of healing, enacted periodically in the coastal villages of Sri Lanka, with mask, costume, and drum. These "Tovil" enactments are both celebration and exorcism for the phantom presences, the spirits of the illnesses that both blight, and perhaps bless—in ways you will learn more about from the book you hold in your hands—our human lives throughout the ages.

Attacked by Poison Ivy is an extraordinary modern excursion into the same territory danced in the Tovil; a revelation of the "mask," the "face" within the psyche, of an illness itself, and its relation to the human quest for selfhood. In this autobiographical narrative, Dr. Ulanov weaves, with a wondrous precision and elegance of language, the tale of her encounter with the mask of a plant-being, a *deva*, or elemental of nature. There are many reasons why this is such a compelling account, inviting our close reading and attention, not only of what "happened" to her, but of her response to illness at a very deep level. Thus this narrative achieves transpersonal relevance: It has something to say to each of us about how to deal with illness, and the limitations and wonderful sensitivity of our physical bodies to inner dialogue.

Ann Ulanov is Johnson Professor of Psychiatry and Religion at Union Theological Seminary, as well as a widely published and renowned Jungian analyst. These levels of accomplishment make her encounter with the elemental being of the *rhus radicans* (poison ivy) both scholarly and insightful. Nor has Ulanov avoided the most intimate kinds of self-analysis and disclosure, making this an exemplary instance of a complex mind deciphering and discovering itself. Ulanov's dialogue with the plant elemental by-passes the *belle naivete* of New Age mythologies, for her counterplayer is not a benign cabbage-enhancing Findhorn deva, rather it is portrayed as a fierce and often inaccessible elemental being, seeming more demon at times than *daimon*, a *nemesis* intent upon testing her in some inscrutable and horrible way. The path to healing lies through the valley of the shadow of illness—this book makes that clear, just as the shamans always taught us. Are we on the trail of an archetype here?

I was privileged to first read the manuscript for this book one late summer, while ill with a bad attack of hay fever, and while my wife Robin lay nearby with the flu. (The two of us were barely able to take care of each other, but we were, in fact, in an ideal state—suffering, immobilized—to experience Ann Ulanov's remarkable chronicle.) Hearing me read aloud passages from the manuscript immediately brought Robin back to her own serious bout with poison ivy years before. I quickly grabbed a note-pad, because what she said was so interesting.

Robin had come from South Carolina to attend graduate school at NYU, and had never really "had" poison ivy before, She had then gone for a weekend outing in the country with friends, which put her in intimate contact with the plant, and about which they had not warned her. (In retrospect, it seemed she might have been rolling in it.) The day after she returned to the city, her body began to itch massively and broke out in red bubbles. Then she began to swell. She became red and stiff, with open running sores, and entered a feverish delirium. She was rushed to the skin clinic at Bellevue hospital in New York, where she remained for over a week, and was even then exhibited to medical students as someone in the very worst categories of responses to poison ivy; where the toxic shock of the reaction becomes almost life-threatening in its intensity. (You have to have experienced this to realize Dr. Ulanov is not at all exaggerating in her account.)

Thereafter Robin became highly allergic to poison ivy, and phobically terrified of encounters anew with the plant.

The mental symptoms of poison ivy, she remembered, were almost worse than the physical. "When I would get it, at the first sign of bumps on the skin I would become panic stricken, anticipating being covered by sores. I had to teach myself not to scratch, but it was awful. The skin would bubble and swell. Often, it burned. I couldn't sleep well, couldn't read or concentrate. I hated my skin, and that feeling soon extended to myself. I didn't want to be seen by anyone, or touched by anyone. The idea was almost unbearable. I guess I somehow felt 'unclean.' As the attack came on, the excruciating panic degenerated into self-loathing and depression."

During this period, Robin went into analysis with Ann Ulanov. "It helped my whole outlook—her (Jungian) ability to look at things symbolically. I was becoming sexually active in those years, and I had a new kind of vulnerability to the body. I wasn't immortal after all. I was becoming a woman, and experiencing incarnation and mortality. The therapy helped to see the nature of any powerful experience, especially illness, as one of being initiated."

Robin and I moved from New York City to a 300-acre farm in the Hudson Valley, where we currently reside. Poison ivy was everywhere, and she was often affected. The dogs and goats wandered in it freely, and even the slightest contact seemed to be disastrous. We began to wonder if it had been a wise decision to move to the country at all.

It was an encounter with an herbalist, Susun Weed, that really helped Robin adjust her attitude. From Weed, Robin learned that poison ivy was more than a "noxious weed" if you will. It was a plant which had an important ecological purpose.

"Susun said that the ivy appeared at the verges of fields cleared for home or roadways or agriculture; especially where men had delved the earth with steel instruments. The ivy was the earth's protective response, a kind of vegetal scar tissue. I began to recognize it as a kind of a warden, a boundary guardian. It encounters you aggressively, and says, 'Are you fit to come here?' I think it was when I first began regarding it as a being, a deva, that things began to change."

During this time I was in training analysis with Dr. Edward Whitmont, a renowned homeopath and Jungian analyst, who also was an important early mentor for Ann Ulanov. With Whitmont's guidance, I began treating Robin homeopathically. We quickly got over the naïve homeopathic fundamentalism (based on a simple "like cures like") that poison ivy itself, *rhus toxicodendron*, would be the right remedy. It simply didn't work. But we found that if we treated the patient and *her* unique experience of the disease—not anybody else's, or what some book says—then she improved. We also learned to work closely with what homeopaths call the "mentals," the psychological complexion of the affliction. "I began to notice that the mental aspects were becoming more formidable," Robin said. "I could tell how strong a poison ivy attack would be by the intensity of the anxiety that preceded it."

We used *anacardium* if she was feeling irritable or angry (uncharacteristic of her) or feeling a sense of unreality; if she was clumsy, stupor alternating with hypervigilance, as well as very swollen, we would use *apis mellifica*, bee toxin. Sometimes sulphur, if she had a headache or sensation of vertigo along with the physical symptoms. We used medium potencies (30c–200c), and the remedies definitely ameliorated the condition once underway, but they did not banish the attacks.

"I stopped all traditional medications, lotions, and ointments, except homeopathy," said Robin. "When the rash started to come on I would only use brown laundry soap, and cool, not warm, water to clean the skin and cut the oils so the rash wouldn't spread. I had to train myself not to scratch. I was talking to it as if it were a being, trying to calm its aggressive guardian energy.

"Walking outside I would admire the beauty and power of the poison ivy plant wherever I saw it. We were now raising dairy goats and milking them. They were not only going into the poison ivy all the time, but they even seemed able to eat it with no apparent ill effect. And I was drinking the milk, which I believe may even have helped to immunize me. I think settling down, farming the land, raising children, also helped to ground me. I became much less reactive.

"But even now when I see the plant, I give it a 'Namaste': 'I recognize and respect the spirit within you. And I ask your permission to walk here in this place, of which you are the guardian.'"

Reading Ann Ulanov's manuscript set each of us off on a profound interior journey—into our own deep resonances with suffering, solitude, meaning, and mortality. A couple of days later Robin and I were both better and engaged in our busy lives, but the reflections remained.

Was the great Sickness-Demon right? Do we need profound encounters with illness and suffering to turn us within? Is the gateway to wisdom an ordeal of suffering? And shall we suffer in silence, like most of our fellow mortals, or wrest from the encounter something of value, and worthy of sharing, because it speaks of the perennial quest of the human soul for meaning?

This book constitutes part of the answer to those questions. As far as good literature is concerned, it certainly seems to help if the mind of the one who suffers illness is as disciplined, textured, and nuanced as Ann Ulanov's. From her ordeal came an exercise in self-examination that is excruciatingly honest and revelatory. It is also luminous and wise. *Attacked by Poison Ivy* provides a prototype for a new kind for inquiry into the mask, or daimon, of an illness. Whatever the kind of the illness, the same process of deepening engagement and dialogue should help. And every human illness invites such an inquiry, because as this book so decisively shows, the implications of such an encounter are always more than medical. They are opportunities to explore the depths of our own natures, and find ourselves to be profoundly spiritual creatures after all.

Attacked by Poison Ivy

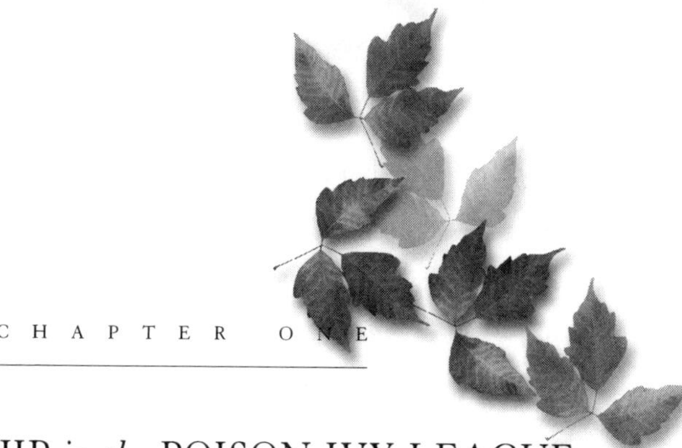

CHAPTER ONE

MEMBERSHIP *in the* POISON IVY LEAGUE

> *It is advisable to approach every illness from the psychological side as well, because this may be extraordinarily important for the healing process. When these two aspects [psyche and physis] work together, it may easily happen that the cure takes place in the intermediate realm . . . that it consists of a* complexio oppositorum, *like the* lapis. *In this case the illness is in the fullest sense a stage of the individuation process.*[1]

WHEN I WAS 50 YEARS OLD, I HAD THE WORST attack of poison ivy I had suffered in four decades. But not *the* worst in my life. That one, when I was about 10, rendered me blind and immobilized for a week during a late hot spring. It took me over a month to recover fully, with eyes swollen shut and encrusted; wrists, ankles, and knees stiff with multiple layers of embedded blisters, armoring me like tiny chains woven so tightly together I could not bend my hands, feet, or legs either backward or forward. I lay unmoving, like a mummy on my bed, encased in searing, itching pain. It made little difference that I couldn't bend, because on the palms of my hands and the soles of my feet lay oblong blisters the size of silver dollars, pulling the skin so tight with trapped juices that I could not bear to stand or hold anything in my hands. Weals covered my legs, back and front, my buttocks, my belly. My chest was blistered. The poison infected my insides, too. My gums puffed, and my inner lips, both above and below, swelled with raw hurt. My ears were scabby, and in their inner chambers myriad tiny blisters crowded together. My knees were bloody from where I had picked off the peeling flesh, and later, when I began to heal, glowed bright pink with new skin. Itching sores crept into my hair, too, and between my fingers and toes. Above all, my body lay weeping, endlessly weeping. The blisters oozed and caked and oozed again. Strips of gauze sopped up some of the fluid, but when removed only ripped the wound open again, so that blood leaked out with serum. I lay in misery, trying to keep still, trying not to stir the air lest it set off new paroxysms of itching.

Ugliness descended, pushing out all beauty, sheathing me completely, as if I had been transmogrified into a gnome. All the senses sent frightful messages. The sounds of itching rose up, like skittering insects racing over the skin, inciting the scrabbly noise of nails digging into skin, the smack of an ankle against a shin, or of one forearm scraping against the other. The smell of sores staining the sheets permeated the bed. The gauze on the wounds glowed with the bright yellow or brown or pink of the different medicines. My skin texture grew tough, like an armadillo, with horny protuberances like a rhino's. My tongue, running over swollen gums and inner cheeks could taste medicinal astringents mixed with leaking, flaking skin, a taste that spoke of lamentation.

The affliction of late November in my 50th year shut one eye; my upper lip stuck out, swollen by two inches, with weals and blisters on my chin, cheek, and neck—disfiguring my face. My breasts, belly, and inner thighs swelled and suppurated with an oily yellow serum. I managed to get an emergency appointment with an allergist who immediately prescribed a massive dose of prednisone, eight pills to be tossed down all at once, reduced only by one pill each day for eight days. This helped, along with oatmeal baths three times during the day, and again in the middle of the night, to quiet the itching so I could sleep, with many applications of alcohol and lotions. My wrists were so stiff with layers of blisters I could not bend them; they required bandaging several times a day to replace the yellowed gauze pads stiff with dried serum.

I remember this ivy episode distinctly because my husband and I were scheduled to lecture two days later at Princeton University, where our youngest son had just entered his freshman year. I called up to warn him, as I knew at his age it was embarrassing just to have parents, let alone one who looked like a troll! Fortunately the prednisone restored my face almost to normalcy, and a long-sleeved blouse with a high neck concealed the rest of my markings. But we had to go early, and I had to stay up late on our return in order to give time to the dressing and redressing of the wounds, to the bathing and medication of the ferocious, burning itch.

The Question

This infection started on a Saturday afternoon when I had gone out for a long walk in the late November autumn splendor. I noticed some itching on Sunday night, but Monday morning really exacted the toll. Seeing my swelling lip and closing eye, and the weals breaking out on my cheek and neck, and feeling a frenzy of itching let loose on the front of my body, I knew I was in serious trouble. I had been there before and recognized the signs which precipitated the emergency call to the doctor.

After seeing the doctor, I went to work to see analysands as scheduled, and continued to work throughout the week. The medication helped, as well as the distraction of focusing intensely on someone else as one does in analytical sessions. I told each person at the beginning of our hour that I was suffering from poison ivy, offering everyone the chance to cancel, lest proximity to me might prompt their own allergic reactions, and because I did look odd. It was at one such telling that something momentous happened, inaugurated by an analysand's question. Himself an analyst, he wondered if I had ever asked myself what my attacks of poison ivy *meant*. His question struck me like a wooden mallet on my forehead. I was stunned.

I had never asked that question, or one even remotely like it, in the fifty years I had been caught by this dread allergy!

And poison ivy had caught me every year of my life, severely as a child, severe only in small patches as an adult. Even with attempts to ward it off, through drops or shots, I became infected, sometimes from the shots or drops themselves. His question stopped me. I realized that in seventeen years of analysis with two separate analysts, and through all the decades of the self-analyzing I had done since, the question had never come up. I had never even thought of it. My analysts had never raised it. My medical doctors had never asked it. This was the first moment such an idea entered consciousness. This hit me as truly remarkable and initiated a long inquiry into this disease and my experiences of it, resulting in writing this book.

The startling realization that the question of the psychological and spiritual meaning of this annual physical suffering had never risen to consciousness brought home to me the reality of the gap employed by dissociated contents to preserve their autonomy. Poison ivy was not a repressed content to me. I could talk about it or share stories of the best treatment for it with friends. I had just never connected it up with my psychic life. I had never received its meaning because, like the fool Parsifal, I never asked the right question.

We work as analysts in analysis. We make our living doing it. But the reality of the psyche, both conscious and unconscious, still unsettles, impresses. All these theories we study and use really are true! For in the moment of my patient's question to me that blank space that heralds a linking up to consciousness of what has been separated, arrested my attention. Blank space arrived, contentless, but resonating with presence. I could physically feel the vibrations of something about to become known, ready to unfold itself.

That blank space is so odd. It is palpably present, but there is just nothing there, only a framed emptiness. As dead air space, a radio that is not broadcasting, but is just about to, alerts our focused attention, I felt myself called to account, to listen. It was singular. Something was connecting; a bridge was crossing a long-held gap. As in Magritte's painting "The Heraclitus Bridge," I saw that under the water, in the unconscious, a bridge had already spanned the river between its two shores, and only above the water, in consciousness, did a gap still loom, waiting for the bridge to be constructed to connect the two sides. I became alert to this gap, to this unknowing, as if I had cat's whiskers extending outward into space. But I needed to wait and know through my body, to receive, to mull, turn over, taste and touch, before any words would arrive.

The Unknown and Theories About It

The stunning presence of something as yet unknown illustrates Wilfred Bion's notion of "beta elements," those undigested experiences in the personality that remain unregistered, unthought. They can occur but are not yet felt; they have not yet reached the status of feelings that require processing by (and in relation to) the rest of the personality. These bits have not yet been transformed into something personal, like an image, a feeling, a thought. They remain circling around in one's psyche, sort of like space-junk. They might manifest themselves as physical pain, or impulsive sex, or even a car crash.[2] In my case, I believe, elements of unprocessed sensuous experience, of pain and sorrow, showed in repetitive bouts of poison ivy.

The reason these elements remain present but undigested, unprocessed by what Bion calls the "alpha function," lies in our wish to avoid unbearable psychic pain. We obliterate such pain by evacuating it in a torrent of speech, or in compulsive actions, and well into the body. One could hazard the guess that poison ivy, too, could be a means to expel unthinkable emotional experience, a physical discharge of unabsorbed psychic events. When my patient asked me what I thought this annual itchy suffering meant, the process began in me to bridge the gap between encapsulated beta bits and my capacity to reach toward them in feeling, thought, and image, setting up resonances between these two distant sides.

A thrumming resonance announced the coming of something. As if hearing annunciation of a future arrival, a coming into being of something new that was not yet there, I felt grasped, summoned to see, to greet, to think about what would be. This state of mind in reference to the specific issue of poison ivy lasted ten years. What arrived was double. Not only did heretofore unknown bits of life (both past and present) make themselves available for living, but a big chunk of subjectivity grew in me with which to entertain them. More "I" arrived that could experience itself thinking, feeling, experiencing what was heretofore unbearable. Not only did this new presence ride into my daily living, but the ass on which it sat—that is, my ability to bear it—grew stronger, more sturdy.

It was the "I" that was not there in the experience of poison ivy. Along with the addition of thinking the unthinkable thought, or feeling the intolerable emotion, arrives a capacity to accept these things, and with it a relation of self to self. This enhanced subjectivity not only can think about and receive the new bits of experience, but can also mull over the processes of thinking itself. Bion believes that the ultimate task of analysis is to introduce patients to themselves.[3]

The discovery of more subjectivity, in addition to the bursting into consciousness of what one had lived but had never joined up with and known about, is an example of Jung's theoretical map of shadow material carrying one's consciousness into the Self. The shadow aspect of my poison ivy experience—its gruesome physical manifestations and impacted psychological emotions—can be seen because it is backlit, illuminated from behind by the larger encompassing Self-dynamics. Just as we ask of a dream presented to our waking ego, "Who took this picture?" so here I was able suddenly to inquire whence comes this yearly affliction, for what purpose does it arrive annually? I saw it in a new light. For Jung, that light emanates from the non-ego perspective of the Self which needs the ego to receive and focus it. That light originates beyond the ego and catches the ego in its glow. I could suddenly see the poison ivy both as coming from somewhere and going somewhere. Bion calls the source and goal of that light "O." For both Bion and Jung the source of that light bestows emotional certainty. I knew now that meaning dwelt in my affliction. I did not know what it was, but I felt its presence would bestow itself on me if I searched and struggled to find it.

I felt opened by my analysand's question. The possibility of meaning advanced from the horizon. The meaning flickered into view and I spent the next decade perceiving it more and more until it flooded me, shedding light that I could now tolerate. It takes us a long time to assimilate a choice for the light. Two dangers loom—that we might over-do and burn out, or under-do out of fear we will burn up. To keep steady, to keep going down into dark places, looking, always looking for the light, builds up a sturdiness to receive what has always been there. The work lies in learning how to take what is offered, to receive what is given, to correspond with luminous grace. That sentimental song we sang as children at camp-fires may sound the right note and also explain why they find it so moving—"Follow the Gleam."

Jung would say that the background light—against which the shadow stuff of poison ivy becomes visible—emanates from and through the Self. Laying hold of the shadow material in this physical affliction can deliver us into the large precincts of Self. We are directed to an ". . . inner process of transformation and rebirth into another being. This 'other being' is the other person in ourselves—that larger and greater personality maturing within us, whom we have already met as the inner friend of the soul. . . . We should prefer to be always 'I' and nothing else. But we are confronted with that inner friend or foe . . . [which one it is] depends on ourselves."[4] For Jung, "healing comes only from what leads the patient beyond herself and beyond her entanglement in the ego."[5]

A choice is necessary. Light is offered, but the road to the light takes us through the ways of pain. Will we choose to face psychic pain? Can we endure working through guilt? Will we "evade frustration or modify it by thought?"[6] Bion's operative word is "thinking." What can be processed by thought will no longer be split-off or dissociated from the rest of the personality.[7] Jung's operative word is "consciousness," and with it the conviction that we will do almost anything to avoid becoming aware of who we are.[8]

Another way to map the arrival of contents hitherto covered up and develop the enhanced subjective capacity to perceive them, can be found in the idea of thinking the "unthought known." Freud noted that loss of a desired object gets converted into an ego loss—we lose that bit of ourselves invested into the object, the loved person. The conflict between that object and the ego can become the space of conversation between the ego's critical activity and the ego now changed by taking the lost object into itself and identifying with it. Christopher Bollas builds on this idea when he reminds us that the ego is social. Built up out of a history of internal relations between the self and other people in our environment, the ego models its relation to the self principally on the parent who transforms our environment to adapt to us when we are infants. The system of caring for us by this "transformational object" becomes a major part of our own self-care system. We know these rules and styles of self-care and self-relating, but we do not rescue them into thought. We are not specifically aware of them. We do them; we do not think them.[9] Like Bion, Bollas believes psychoanalysis brings this unthought known into consciousness through the relationship between analysand and analyst.[10] In my case, poison ivy encapsulated a long series of interactions between me, my body, those caring for me, and, in Jungian terms, what was reaching me from a non-ego transcendent point of origin. This condensed lump of the unthought known repeated itself once a year for almost fifty years. Only in the decade that followed could I rescue it into thought, process it into feeling, come to know what I did not know I had known, but what had known me.

Such a discovery, or recovery, is like a small resurrection. It was something that had lived itself over and over again in varying degrees of intensity in my body, and it now became available to be lived consciously. Jung sees correctly here. Consciousness makes all the difference. What was entombed in repetitive suffering becomes released into living, and the body is right in the center of it. On the one hand, from a direction of descent from above to below, from ego to unconscious, things that should have been consciously apprehended fell, instead, into the concrete body. This false incarnation made literal what should have been symbolic, displaced into the body to act out what the ego would not admit and process. As Jung says, "such suspended ideas can express themselves easily in the body, in certain skin troubles, for instance."[11] On the other hand, in the opposite direction, ascending upward from the underground, from unconscious to conscious, my body was repeatedly speaking about a pattern of experience that was striving to be recognized in image, thought, feeling, and dream. The body repeatedly made its point, itself being the agent of a consciousness not located in the ego, a somatic consciousness that supports and promotes the smaller light of the ego. Jung writes, "the physiological unconscious, the so-called somatic unconscious which is the subtle body . . . becomes material, because the body is the living unit, and our conscious and unconscious are embedded in it."[12] Just as through everyday consciousness we receive intimations of immortality, just so, through the subtle body of somatic consciousness, we receive bulletins of something beyond the ego. This "something" transmits an awareness of the greater field of energy encompassing us, originating outside us yet directly addressing us.

In this experience we enter the precincts of something known in the body but still to be known in the mind. That ancient psychologist Augustine discusses this transition in terms of time and self-knowledge. Chronological time, he says, is a succession of events that allows us to distinguish past, present, and future; it builds narrative sequence that allows us to tell our story to each other and to ourselves. In contrast, present and eternal time, he says, comprise a simultaneity of events that occur in a sort of primordial moment where all that is, all that belongs to reality, is right here, now. In such moments, it is as if for an instant we broke through historical, chronological narrative time to the transcendent *now*, to *is*-ness. We see the whole of which we are a part. In the case of my poison ivy attacks, in such moments I could see the larger reality to which they belonged—how they were both a speaking out and a substitute for speech, both a manifestation and a covering, a narrative of my personal past and an annunciation of what sought to break free of those tangled relationships. I think of Emily Dickenson's splendid line: "Behind this mortal bone / There knits a Bolder one."[13]

In the moment of being asked about the meaning of annual poison ivy attacks, the meaning they possessed arrived. It took me quite a while to catch up to the revelation, to grasp what had grasped me. Augustine helps in that process with his understanding of the *memoria* that enlarges our sense of memory. *Memoria* includes both our senses of time, the narrative and the *nunc stans*, all our moments of eternal now. When we resort to *memoria*, we enter a storehouse of experience and look around. Here we retain human experience in the mind, storing traces of sense-perception and what we have made of them. Jung calls this the realm of archetypes, self-portraits of the instincts, which express themselves in primordial images of human instinct, images that support and transgress the human ego.[14] Time and timelessness thus intersect in and through each of us, as well as around and beyond us. We experience Augustine's two kinds of time, one that abides forever, outside time, bestowing on us perception of the simultaneity of events; and the other that is immediate, here-and-now succession of events and thoughts.[15] In psychoanalytic terms, this intersection can be described as the meeting of our historical past, the past of our individual object relations, with the shared, collective, human past, recorded in repeated and timeless human images of the basic patterns of human existence—mother, father, child, journey, goal.

Augustine goes further to say explicitly that in the depths of the self, through *memoria*, we behold, in addition to patterns of human experience, the image of God—who is creator of all time. Augustine thus links the depth of human self to God, matching a small trinity of memory, understanding, and will to the inseparable threeness and oneness that compose the ultimate unity and multiplicity in God.[16] Augustine says of God as Trinity, "It is, it beholds, it loves."[17] In our triad of being, knowing, and loving, we are bid to return to ourselves and make our way back to the Trinity, for "There our being will meet no death, our knowledge no mistaking, our loving no failure."[18] Thus Augustine makes explicit the source of light that creates and expands our subjectivity and bestows emotional certainty upon us. When we enter *memoria*, we are both reached by and reach back to the presence of God.

The mind made in the image of God remembers, understands, and loves God in loving itself, and when it loves God also loves its neighbor.[19] In relation to the all-too-human problem of poison ivy, this means that recovering to awareness what was condensed, conserved, left in the shadow realm of undigested beta experience, and the unthought known now also opens up the self to that which transcends it, authors it, and anchors it. Jung calls our image of that presence the Self, which I understand as that in us which is not God but knows about God, and indeed makes a bridge to the transcendent, in whatever guise we apprehend it.

Now over a decade later, I can put into words what I have discovered. As is usual with such blank space, when something experienced but unknown grants itself to be more known, one doubts its veracity. Maybe I am once again making mountains out of molehills, magnifying, exaggerating, or even malingering. All the theories I have learned crowd in—this is hysterical excess, projection, overdetermination. No doubt there is some measure of truth in all of these accusations. But as any sufferer of the ravages of the poisonous sumac, oak, or ivy can attest, this compounding of pain and itching, of blood and serum, of scarring and raw nerve endings, amounts to massive body-grief. What brought home its reality to me—the horror of the pain—was my husband's reaction to my moanings when lowering myself into the bath, to feel the hot water exacerbate the itching to fever pitch, or cauterize the bleeding sores. He couldn't stand it, just hearing me! Sometimes he went to the other end of the apartment. His amazement, and compassion, at the extent of what this allergy inflicted brought home to me that my suffering was real, that what I felt was painful, and that my sounds were my witness of its reality.

From my husband's response, I learned that we need to be witnessed to feel real, that another's beholding and attesting grants value to what we experience. Even prayer cries out with this "yearning for witnessed significance," as the Psalms show.[20] I suddenly remembered then a rhythmic jingle I had composed at age 10, in the most terrible of my ivy attacks. I could recall the words and the tune came back to me, too, as I saw myself lying on my back holding one of my knees, singing to its bleeding cuts and pustulent wounds. I witnessed my body's hurt, filling in the absence of anyone else's presence.

More Questions

Recalling the jingle brought other questions. Why did I contract poison ivy every year of my life? Why were the regimens of medicinal drops or shots ineffective in preventing recurrence of the outbreak of this allergy? Why was I never stopped from going into places at my country home where the lush ivy proliferated? Most important of all, why was it that every time poison ivy beset me it was as if it were the first time? Why did my body have no memory?

I knew poison ivy was not classified as a psychosomatic disease, but rather a contact allergy. This means that the best prevention is to avoid contact, to remove oneself from even a distant proximity to the infectious plant. But for someone like me, who as a child could contract the allergy even from the air, especially if poison ivy were being burned in the fall clean-up of leaves, or could succumb to its oil just from passing by its growth on the side of the road, avoidance was all but impossible to achieve. Poison ivy grows luxuriantly and persistently in ditches, woods, fields, in brush, up trees, in sandy places, on rocky paths, along walls and fences. It grows in family garbage and town dumps. It grows wild, without human care. It grows in trailing fashion along the ground, and ascends to an abundant blooming, winding around trees, producing lush foliage that stands forth like a tree on its own. Poison ivy returns despite conscientious spraying with herbicides or strenuous efforts to uproot it. Its beauty includes tiny, shiny, bright red-green leaves as it buds in the spring, turning a lustrous dark green in large foliage through the summer, turning again deep crimson, gold, and purple in the autumn. It bears clusters of berries that resemble the pale gray beauty of bayberry with the coming of winter. Indeed it was just those berries that proved my downfall that late November. I thought they were bayberries and plucked some bunches for the house!

That, too, struck me as extraordinary (after my patient put his question to me). Why didn't I know the property of this deadly enemy to beguile through its alluring berries? How could I not have known, not have studied its multiform presentations? Had I learned nothing from my yearly suffering of its attacks? Clearly, I was a victim of neglect—my own, and that of others about me to forewarn me as a child and prevent me where possible against contact with the ivy—but also the neglect accompanying poison ivy itself. It grows in abandoned areas; it thrives on being overlooked, disregarded, untended. It grows wild. It flourishes by the side of the road and in refuse. I contracted an allergy to what was neglected, untended, and rejected. Or, to put it psychodynamically, my psyche made use of this overlooked, abandoned plant to arouse my system to express my own experiences of neglect. Like the *prima materia* of alchemy, that indefinable basic stuff which energies and processes transform into the precious *lapis* stone, poison ivy was "cheap as dirt . . . the most despised and rejected thing, 'thrown out into the street,' 'cast on the dunghill,' . . . 'found in filth.'"[21] It got under my skin and became a crucial episode, or "operation," in an alchemical sense: "In this case the illness is in the fullest sense a stage in the individuation process."[22]

Another astonishing fact came to light after the attack that occurred when I was 50. I realized I had never dreamed of poison ivy. I discovered this because now, for the first time in my life, it did turn up in my dreams. They helped me uncover in images (and then in words) what had been going on in this recurring physical event in my life. Somatic consciousness—what my body reenacted—taught me much more than I had known before about body-speech. Even more surprising to me, *astounding* really, is the fact that I have not had a major attack of poison ivy since inquiring into its psychic and spiritual meaning.

Well, just one little attack, a small ivy-bout when, five years after the big one at 50, I did to myself what I discovered had been done to me: I neglected myself. I refused to take care; I could not be bothered to take minimal precautions when in the neighborhood of the green ivy leaves. I was too lazy to put on long trousers and bind the cuffs at wrist and ankle. With a cavalier attitude, I persisted in clearing out that patch of brush. Mind would triumph over the matter of what the garlands of shiny green heralded. I did not take care to wash in a preventive liquid soap after returning indoors. I paid the price and saw immediately that I had inflicted on myself once again what benign neglect had repeatedly jeopardized me with in the past. My neglect to care for myself brought into awareness a memory of being forgotten and overlooked, time and time again throughout my childhood. Indeed, the ivy that blooms in neglect, that is never cared for except to exterminate it, joined with the human neglect of the person—myself. We intertwined.[23]

Aims

My questions and discoveries invited me to interpret this allergy as if it were in fact psychosomatic. I accepted this adventure with the following goals compelling my attention. The impact of this contact allergy is intensified by its psychic reality, to which I did not pay attention, nor did anyone else. In my researches, I have found that doctors and chemists are tone deaf to the fact that the psyche of the sufferer may be contributing to the potency of the affliction. A first aim, then, is to speak for myself and all others of the poison-ivy tribe—my Ivy League—to mount a sort of class-action suit for consciousness in those who deal with the allergy as physical only, and only under the microscope, omitting the contributions of heart, mind, and soul. The American Academy of Dermatology claims that the poison plants of ivy, sumac and oak "are the single most common cause of allergic reactions in the United States and will affect ten to fifty million Americans every year" a number which matches the proportions of great cities of people, all suffering poison ivy![24]

Poison ivy is like the common cold. We know many suffer from it, but there it is, not much to be done about it. I disagree. Much can be done if we use the resources of the psyche to deal with an allergy that is not, strictly speaking, psychogenic. The body-speech of its many sufferers reaches enough volume to invite professionals to tune in to this allergy psychologically as well as physically. The purpose of such examination is to reduce the misery, especially of the children (who number poison ivy's chief victims), and their parents, who might then take precautions and expand preventive measures to spare their little ones this torment. Both sufferers and professionals treating and researching the condition may then learn about an illness which, at bottom, is an immunological one. Diseases of the immune system we know will prove central to the 21st century. Perhaps this trivial but vexing allergy, reaching us in its neglect from the side of the road, will prove to be the stone the builders rejected, contributing a small but decisive foundation to treat all attacks on the body's immune system.

A second aim concerns the process of analysis itself. The difference investigating its psychological meaning made to my contracting the allergy astounded me. Something uttered only in body-speech, when inquired into could be rescued into dream-images, through which poured great affect, which then could be translated into words. The body had conserved in suffering the meaning of many layers of experiences willingly yielding to a multiple discourse of affect, image, thought, and word—that is, once my consciousness asked, sought, waited, listened, and finally heard. That those multiple languages stopped all further physical attacks brought not only incredible physical relief, but wonder at the power of analysis. It really made a difference, even when restricted to the process of self-analysis, which is harder than analyzing another person because of our inevitable blind spots. Analysis equips us to converse with the mad parts of ourselves—the mute parts, the left-out parts. The willingness of the psyche to make known from body to affect, to image, to thought, to action (or the ceasing of action, no more allergic reaction), is deeply impressive. Such a happening makes us aware of how important it is that the ego take an attitude of humble inquiry, joining with the body to assemble meaning from conversations at a deep level between body, mind, heart, and soul.

This intercession of consciousness also instructs us in the power of the body itself. Body-speech is not only to be translated "upward" into words. Our body communicates eloquently in its own terms, even better than in words, because body-symbolism is big enough to capture the spirit as well as the physical fact. My body expressed the meaning of suffering I found and created in poison ivy. But words and feelings surprised me, and also conferred a great boon on me. Words led me to a different space where I was allowed to relinquish the excesses of annual physical suffering. Even more, this space ushered me into a truth in living that could not be grasped in words.

I hope, then, to demonstrate the power of analysis, both in recovering the past so it can be realigned into the present, as well as looping the present into the past. Both past and present then change. The present grows down into the past to gain new roots there; and the past reaches up to bloom anew in the present. This linking of past and present produces not only a clarifying linear causality, it also permits us to step outside causality, out of historical determinism into the presence of an originating meaning that comes to address us. Meaning has already assembled through intensity of affect conserved through bodily states.

Memory piled on memory: the harsh smell and grainy texture of Fels Naptha laundry soap used to scrub the skin clean of the poisonous resin, followed by the mollifying liquid of calamine lotion, which seemed to be scented pale pink, like its color; the cooling touch of fine linen sheets, changed often to bring relief from secreting sores; the dappled patterns of light on the ceiling, whether from eyes stuck shut or curtains half drawn against the afternoon heat; the hushed humming of insects outside the open windows and muted noises from the kitchen or library within the house. These bodily memories all speak of how much we experience through the flesh, without words, before and after words. Words are not the only way to communicate; they are not always available, nor necessarily the best way to communicate. The recovery of so much body-experiencing rolled in like the sea, one wave after another, seemingly endless, bringing the richness of a child's perceptive and apperceptive abilities. All that stored-up life surged in me, drenching the present.

Such a flood of memories conjoined past and present, and also opened the future, even moving into the future, bringing release from physical suffering, and opening up time itself. As Dōgen, the 13th-century Buddhist, saw, time is neither out of time beyond moments, nor is it an endless series of moments. Each moment lived fully reveals a crossroad of times.[25] Analysis *now* of what had happened *then* joins the then and now, yielding precious information about those I had loved as a child—those who had loved me and where we had failed to meet and match—thus providing a great deal of "object relations" history. This organ-dialect of a body enduring poison ivy gave yearly voice to the suffering and effort to heal it in myself and in my family.

Analysis also grants vision of the archetypal energy of the psyche, and with it, our construction of symbols to express the meaning of that energy as we encounter it in our personal lives. In this conjunction of physical and psychical, of event and meaning, of personal and archetypal symbol, we find and create a spiritual universe. Dōgen speaks of "time-being"[26] where each moment carries all of time, and all that is real is here and now. The timeless moment also locates us in space; the self is located in the stillness of all movement. What declares itself for our reception is the truth as "endless, unremitting, unthinkable, unnameable."[27]

Only this reality that transcends our specific time and space meets the unthinkable primitive agonies that befall us before our ego is formed and resilient enough to metabolize them for use in living. We feel beset by psychotic anxieties—about falling forever, about fragmenting and never cohering to take up residence in our very own body, or about failing to connect with external objects, so that we end up living as if cocooned in fantasies floating in outer space, or entombed in factual reality without any balm of imaginative living.[28] Such agonies leave us resourceless to face transcendent reality, the reality that transcends our egos.

Those early anxieties leave gaps in our egos; we carry the resultant dissociations into our adult lives. When we attempt intimacy—with another person, with a profound idea, with a political ideal, with an imaginative image, with a religious vision—those gaps present their bill. They seek integration. By then, however, the specific childhood environment and the persons who peopled it no longer exist in our daily lives as mother and father, sister and brother, as they once did. The terms of integration must be conjugated in a different grammar. Nor can we—if we succeed in facing the breakdowns that have already happened, in the past—just blame those who hurt us by doing something awful to us, or by failing to do something loving with us. We see through our wounds to the wounds of others. That leads us inevitably to the reality that undergirds and transcends all of us, and to the great theological questions of why evil prospers, why terrible things afflict people.

Our primitive dissociations—for which we can find no words or images—meet up with a transcendent reality whose language surpasses words and images. Its language of silence seems too much like those primitive holes in our ego where unthinkable unprocessed anxieties assaulted us. Only as our egos mend and metabolize these primordial fears can we differentiate their void and abyss from the Vast and All of the transcendent. We need an intermediary ego to process the meetings with both our primitive anxieties and the overwhelming presence of the transcendent.

Our body-speech begins out of two opposite experiences: our experience of primordial agony that leaves gaps of dissociation in our egos, and our experience of the untranslatable procession of the infinite toward our small finite awareness. The psyche and the body together collaborate to witness and express what is happening. The psyche makes use of the dialect of bodily organs to communicate the experience we undergo—whether it be sublime or abysmal, for both defy words and images. To recover such experiences to the communicable forms of words and images, we do not just discard body-speech, as if translating beyond it to a superior mode. Instead, we increase our capacity to listen, to engage and disengage our ego skills, to see through them as we use them to move into the speech of the spiritual universe that communicates the meanings of even such *lowly* paltry experiences as recurrent allergies.

The body can speak of such truth in a way our words fail to do. Our body captures direct immediate experience, knowing more than the conventional mind and intellect. Pertinent to my encounter with poison ivy are Dōgen's words: "When you discuss 'outside,' skin, flesh, bones, and marrow are all outside. When you discuss 'inside,' skin, flesh, bones, and marrow are all inside."[29] Poison ivy took me into another realm, where opposites dwelt side by side, to Jung's *complexio oppositorum*: liminal and boundaried space, assertion and submission, abandonment and meeting, mute illness and speaking true from the heart. The moment opened up, and returned these many years later in its open, unblocked form to my surface mind, hauling up with it the anchor to the depths. Thus I could follow the chain of associations down to the root of my suffering, while also releasing myself from it. Poison ivy functioned for me as a true *prima materia*, as the *radix ipsius*, "root of itself," by introducing me to that which is, in itself, both author and goal.

Not until I finished this project did I see that it demonstrated what can happen in a self-analysis. Significant questions for all those engaged in analysis, whether as analysand or analyst, are: "After analysis, what? Do we change in a way so deep that it continues in us as a new bit of reality in which we live, that lives in us? Or is analysis, finally, a phase of self-help that fades with the passing years?" Because of this study of poison ivy, I see that what I believe about the efficacy of analysis is really what I do believe. Analysis aims to establish and strengthen a vibrant inner conversation between psyche and self, between surface and depth mind, between all the parts—conscious, unconscious, somatic, spiritual, psychological, mental. That conversation is what changes us—for good, pun intended. That inner conversation seeds connection to all the parts of our outer world—other bodies, the bodies politic and social, the cultural body, the mystical body, thus including neighbors both near and far, both present and past, and into the future.

I wish, then, to rescue the *rhus radicans* from neglect, and to contribute to the healing of its attacks by beginning with the somatic facts about this allergy (chapter 2). Memory reveals an intricate object relations history in my repeated exposure to this affliction. We see afresh the usefulness for the analysis of psychosomatic conditions of the facts of dependency and the power of body-speech to communicate emotions not yet imaged or verbalized (chapter 3). Poison ivy, of all things—this neglected weed—constellates archetypal conjunctions that bring into "being-time" the still-point through which reality always offers itself with spirit and meaning (chapter 4). This study illustrates the possibility of what comes after analysis—living the reality to which that inner conversation going on in all of us bears witness (chapter 5).

CHAPTER TWO

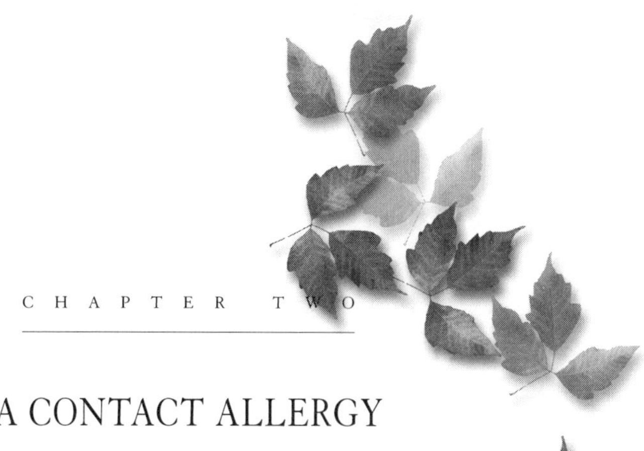

A CONTACT ALLERGY

A wrong functioning of the psyche can do much to injure the body, just as, conversely, a bodily illness can affect the psyche; for psyche and body are not separate entities but one and the same life.[1]

POISON IVY IS CLASSIFIED IN DERMATOLOGY AS A contact allergy. Contact allergies, by definition, are not psychosomatic. In researching books on psychosomatic medicine, this devilish allergy rarely rates any mention at all because it is thought to be devoid of psychogenic origin. The very classification points to its source: if no contact occurs, one is spared the reaction.

That is all true. One does not manufacture the symptoms out of psychic stuff, nor originate the signs of infection without exposure to the plant. For years, there was little to be done for its cure except to stay out of the plant's way to prevent becoming infected; or, if one succumbed, then wait it out, using the soap, the baths, the lotions. Recovery usually takes about three weeks, though that follows the eight to forty-eight hours for the contact to bloom on the skin. Once infected, the time to return to health extends to a month, if not more.[2]

Some doctors I consulted refused to give shots or drops because they found it a nuisance to acquire the serum when the results proved so unreliable. In addition, the shots were extremely painful. The injection of the poison serum, based in alcohol, felt like a continuing penetration of the needle going on and on into one's deepest insides. Along with leaving painful lumps on my arm, the shots often produced a thick patch of infection that needed to be bandaged for several weeks. Trying the shots deep in the buttock, at a doctor's suggestion, proved even worse. It set off convulsive itching far under the skin. Instead of blisters leaking down my arm, my haunch inwardly exploded in frenzied irritation that could not be reached, making me want to take a hair brush to the outer skin in an effort to transmit relief to the inside paroxysms. The medicinal drops were no better. The prescription was to take 1 drop three times a day in a full glass of water, increasing the dose by 1 drop each day, up to 15 drops, and then daily decreasing them back down to 1 drop. Midway along the dosage, I felt as if my veins were itching, as if my throat and stomach were erupting into a radically excitable pruritis. Doctors advised, "You can't prevent it; when you catch it, just put up with it." The disease itself suffers from neglect! Patients are abandoned.

Nonetheless, the question arises as to why some of us react so severely and others fly off scott free. Both are exposed; only one is afflicted. What consigns some of us to life-membership in the Ivy League? Why do some of us react to each subsequent exposure as if we possessed no immune system at all? My sister, for example, came down with one bad bout of the ivy disease, but thereafter grew some inner protection against it, so that if it recurred at all, it did so only in minor degrees, despite her frequent exposure to the vine while riding her horse. My agitated response posed the crucial questions: "Why does the body fling itself into massive defense every time as if it is the first time? Where was body memory? What interfered with the body's immune system?" I was hunting for the unknown X.

Growing in waste places, *rhus radicans* (*rhus rydbergia*) is poisonous in all its parts (except the pollen grains), even in winter, and in both wet or dry places.[3] It thrives in all fifty of the United States, but along with poison sumac (*rhus vernix*) and poison oak (*rhus diversiloba*) is limited to North America, including Canada and northern Mexico.[4] Poison ivy and poison oak have been introduced to Japan, and to Europe, where the vines have been trained for ornament and to help bolster the dykes in the Netherlands. It belongs to an international botanical Anacardiaceae family, which includes the pistachio nut, cashews, mangos, and the Japanese lacquer tree, all of which are found in Japan, China, India, and Burma, and in tropical regions, such as Hawaii and Central America.[5] Poison ivy produces allergic reactions in the skin of all those who are sensitive to it. Studies vary in estimating how many of a population may be susceptible to being conscripted into the Ivy League. One out of two people is allergic to some degree, and some are so severely allergic that hospitalization is required.[6] Other studies say approximately 85 percent of the population in the United States "will develop an allergic reaction if exposed to poison ivy." And 10 to 15 percent of the population (that is twenty-five to forty million people!) are thought to be "extremely susceptible to poison ivy."[7]

How Allergies Work

The formula reads: *Rhus* = PI PO PS phenols, all of which contain widely allergenic oleoresin and urushiol, which are composed of a mixture of compounds, the worst being phenolic resin, pentadecylcatechol.[8] These compounds produce severe dermatitis, large blisters, lesions, swelling, pruritis, headache, fever.[9] In addition, if the reaction is acute, it causes an edema that is intercellular and, if severe, will lead to vesiculation (inflammation and circumscribed elevation of the epidermis containing serous fluid), acanthosis (thickening of the epidermal layer), parakeratosis (a disorder affecting the horny layer of the epidermis), and exocytosis (inflammation entering epidermis).[10] The resin can easily seep out of the plants and be transferred to the fur of dogs, cats, horses; indeed, to most pets, as well as to shoes, clothing, firewood, gardening tools, fishing rods, and the like. Fast action is needed—within 5 to 10 minutes after contact—washing with water and detergent soap, because the oleoresin quickly gets under the skin's surface and can result in a chemical spread to body sites not directly exposed to the plant. New lesions can break out as long as three weeks after the initial exposure. The allergy makes working, sleeping, and even just surviving, a challenge. Repeated attacks do not confer immunity. No accepted method of immunization has evolved.[11]

Poison ivy is classified as a Hypersensitivity Type IV contact allergy. White blood cells that fight infection, known as lymphocytes, are divisible into two major kinds: B cells and T cells. Both act to confer immunity on the body. B cells provide humoral immunity, so called because it circulates in the bloodstream. B cells are activated in lymph nodes and spleen to manufacture antibodies to fight off invaders, called antigens. In poison ivy, it is T cells, activated in the thymus gland, which produce lymphokines, which stimulate macrophages (scavenger cells) to attack the antigens (the invading oil of poison ivy) directly within the cells rather than by producing antibodics. The immunity provided by the T cells is called cell-mediated because it takes place within or on the cell. The T cells (and the B cells) remember the attacker, the antigen they have battled, and are prepared to act if the invader attacks again.

To sum up the process of infection again, it begins when the urushiol oil contained in poison ivy comes in contact with the skin and an eczematous reaction sets in. The "immunologically active portions of the agents . . ." [that is, the urushiol oil of the plant] are called "haptens." Too small to be antigenic themselves, the haptens "penetrate the epidermis and conjugate . . .

to body proteins,"[12] which bind to Langerhans' cells, derived from bone marrow, and located in the epidermis. The Langerhans' cells serve in the epidermis as antigen-presenting-cells, whereas in the dermis, the macrophage (scavenger cells) serve that purpose. The antigen-presenting-cells then enter the regional lymph nodes, "where the antigen is processed and presented to the CD4 + T lymphocytes."[13] The T lymphocytes release "immunostimulatory cytokines."[14] The cells then react to the allergen, the invading oil, and fight it after first showing the clinical symptoms of rash, swelling, blisters, inflammation, and itching. The rash spreads, not because of the fluid leaking from the blisters, but instead, from the traces of urushiol on fingernails or clothing, or outdoor equipment. The urushiol shows remarkable tenacity.

Antihistamine drugs to block the body's overproduction of the inflammatory histamine, like prednisone (and its variants, such as doxycycline), are now used for poison ivy among many other afflictions. Prednisone suppresses symptoms, but suppression is no cure, as anyone taking it knows, because when we stop taking the drug, the symptoms recur, though in a much less drastic form. I found with poison ivy that the blisters, though much less virulent, came alive again once I finished the dosage of medicine.

The skin barrier proves for the Ivy Leaguer remarkably sensitive, indeed hyper. The usual meanings for hypersensitive include touchy, emotional, temperamental. And the enemy, the urushiol, proves a fierce antagonist. The battle waged against the invader occurs within the body cells, within the units of our physical life. The invasion reaches deep and mobilizes a kind of recognition, somatically, of what has attacked before, and stimulates immune responses, to combat the invader and to assemble once again a protective barrier, a resistant covering, a safe, clear, free shell within which to live, made unsusceptible to the poisonous infiltrator.[15] But this contact sensitivity results in a chemical (the dread urushiol oil of poison ivy) being absorbed through the skin that proves stronger than the skin barrier. Once inside, the cell "memory" combats the invader once again, but a kind of somatic unconsciousness, or naiveté, keeps letting the invasion occur.

Why does the Ivy Leaguer have to do this again and again? Has the memory within the cells lapsed? Is the skin hyper-permeable? Could we say on a somatic level that some kind of insulation within our own skin has not been achieved by the Ivy Leaguer? Instead, we remain highly impressionable to the surroundings, to what drifts in the air, and originates from something still growing despite efforts to destroy it, with deep roots almost impossible to plough up. Resources to defend do get mobilized, but are insufficient to daunt the invader at first threat. Each time it is a cycle of contact, invasion, spreading of infection, counterdefense, and eventual healing, but only after some weeks pass. A repetition occurs, and reoccurs; no insurance is built up against future menace, no accumulation of memory repels repeated invasion. We could almost imagine an individual disposition which makes use of the environment to pull the individual downward to reach consciousness of what lies below the surface.[16]

False Conjunction of Opposites

What is striking is that in the Ivy Leaguer's body the opposites of invasion and defense do not relate or combine in the right way. Instead, a sort of fusion occurs. The oil infiltrates and the body ingests it—sucks it up. Only then does a battle ensue. In the symbolic terms of alchemy, these elements produce a false or "lesser conjunction" of opposites that wreak havoc in the body, leading to "contamination and death," instead of to a true joining which issues in greater unity and equilibrium.[17] The body-ego, so to speak, is knocked out, succumbing to a long painful *mortificatio* of poison ivy that must simply be endured until its end, like a "dark night of the body,"[18] in the darkened room where I lay almost blind for a week. Sufficient distance and discrimination between the opposites has not been established. The body-ego is weak here, not sufficiently asserting its integrity, symbolized by the skin container to protect the inside and act as a barrier against an outside poisonous penetrator. The body-ego needs to develop the ability to recognize the danger, and assert its own protective barricade.

To reach a true joining of opposites, in what alchemists call the "greater conjunction," a stable and durable body-consciousness must be established by adequately differentiating its antagonists into discrete entities that confront each other. Poison ivy sufferers need the reliable somatic consciousness that the nonallergic body possesses, in place of personal hypersensitivity and permeability. We need, so to speak, to stand up for ourselves and not allow in what will poison us. Space must be created between the opposites for somatic consciousness to strengthen, to wake up to the danger of the insidious poison ivy oil.

The "lesser *coniunctio* . . . refers to a premature union of insufficiently separated opposites," a kind of "unconscious incest . . . an unconscious incestuous longing for containment in the mother." A person afflicted by poison ivy suffers from skin that no longer functions as an adequate container, but skin that is gouged, leaking, broken up, even shattered. Such a "lesser *coniunctio*," the "living out of unconscious incest tendencies, is always followed by a catastrophe."[19]

Somatic Consciousness and Space

With somatic consciousness—a body-awareness comparable to ego-consciousness, where we really know what we are doing and where we are physically—the elements achieve discrete and distinct existence and confront each other, eventually to join in right measure and order. In alchemy, such a true conjoining of opposites produces the *lapis*, the Philosopher's Stone, symbolizing a new center, hard as rock, consolidating both a personal and transpersonal experience of reality.

With the intercession of consciousness, initiated by my analysand's question about the meaning of my repeated attacks of poison ivy, the door opened to venture toward such adamantine knowledge. I began to learn what poison ivy attacks symbolized for me, persistently, repeatedly attacking me until I sought to "'redeem' that which has metamorphosed into physical disease . . . [to] envision the process as a 're-sublimation' of something that has fallen victim to materialization."[20] The body space needed between the opposites of my hyper-sensitivity and the oil's too persistent poisoning shows similarities to Winnicott's transitional space.[21]

In transitional space, which Winnicott describes in reference to infants, the child moves from dependence on its mother to find and create its very own self and the symbols that represent the unity it has known with its parent. The child effects this growth into self and symbolic life through play. The adult goes on using transitional space to feed and deepen self and symbol through the play-space of culture.[22] For chronic poison-ivy-sufferers, the transitional space between the inner self and the outer world—the body container and the environment surrounding it—are not sufficiently differentiated as separate realms interacting with each other. Here the poisonous plant seeps into a vulnerable body.

Somatic consciousness arises from the differentiation of opposite elements, not their fusion, and not from one invading and canceling the other. The body-self must distinguish the correct proportion of threat and protection, as well as the outer from the inner reality. Separating what is harmful from what is helpful increases body discretion, implying an adaptive "body-sight" that sees the leaves of the poison ivy plant out there, and vulnerability in here under the skin, and a space between them. Members of the Ivy League must effect a kind of alchemical *separatio*.[23]

In psychodynamic terms, the Ivy Leaguer gets caught in repetition compulsion *on the body level*. Here we distinguish not just the hypersensitivity of the body and the powerful intruding urushiol in poison ivy plants, we must also discern soul need and body need. Their separation—that is, their differentiation—must take place. Otherwise, the body is forced into repeatedly acting out physically what is also a psychic invasion—fighting off infection from the environment. Chronic itching and scratching on a symbolic level "heralds the opening of the spirit world." Etymologically, the word "scratch" stems from the root *greb*, which in German relates to *graben,* "to dig," as in digging up, sorting through, meditating and ruminating.[24] The soul's need I will take up in chapter 3.

The needed development of somatic consciousness, like finding and creating a personal body-self in relation to the world, is analogous to Winnicott's description of a child's finding and creating consciousness of a personal self in relation to others, under the protection of the mother's holding the space for the child at first, and then reflecting back to the child within that space the budding self of the child.[25] Repeated severe afflictions of poison ivy can be seen as a wrecking of the transitional space for both body and mind. The potential space does not firmly establish itself, but gets invaded and poisoned, so that we are not "held," nor "reflected back." We do not develop symbols of the self's experience coming into being as a psychosomatic unity in relation to the world.[26] Repair includes re-establishing that space where an Ivy Leaguer can make the transition from self to world, from dependence to independence, equipped with real symbols that disclose both psychic and bodily reality.

C. G. Jung also looks to the space between physis and psyche for the cure of somatic affliction: "When these two aspects work together, it may easily happen that the cure takes place in the intermediate realm . . . that it consists of a *complexio oppositorum*, like the *lapis*."[27] He extends the opposites even to characterizing the nature of God. True opposites are not totally contrary because "they do show a constant propensity to union." Because they are opposites, "they form a potential." He finds the extreme poles of spirit and instinct to be "one of the commonest formulations," with "the advantage of reducing the greatest numbers of the most important and complex psychic processes to a common denominator." Thus "psychic processes seem to be balances of energy flowing between spirit and instinct. . . . Psychic processes therefore behave like a scale along which consciousness 'slides.'"[28] With reference to my poison ivy attacks, the "spiritual" aspects of the condition were subordinated to the body's instinctual response. The opposites collided and one subsumed the other, thus causing the body to reiterate its spiritual distress annually. Healing can be seen as inviting consciousness to "slide" toward the spiritual pole and thus to restore the space of "potential." That incipient potency was what I felt as the arrival, yet unformulated either in dream image, word, or symbol, of the presence of meaning. This whole essay is my effort to woo meaning into a visible form that communicates to me, and to others, its curative power.

A psychological parallel to this emphasis on the "space between" as a source of healing comes from the completely different voice of Jacques Lacan, who claimed he was returning to the origins of the origins, to the Ur-Freud. For Lacan, the effectiveness of therapy comes about by the analyst and the analysand achieving "the correct distance."[29] That distance describes the proper space between the analytic couple, as well as between consciousness and unconsciousness in both doctor and patient, and, as well, the just distance from truth itself. For truth can never be spoken whole, but only through "Mid-dire"—mid-speak—in order to capture appropriately the reversals, negations, negations of negation, and just coming to be of the new in the unconscious."[30] The alternatives are many and various. We can fall into identification with all the identities imposed upon us at birth—legal, familial, cultural, national—at the cost of our unique identity, and resulting in the neurotic state that brings the analysand to analysis in the first place. Or, we can take the option of madness, where we succumb to the archaic chaos of inundating reality. Or we can choose the option of the mystic who knows that love exists and that it "depends on God's *jouissance*." Lacan says, "The mystical ejaculations are neither idle chatter nor inane verbiage but . . . the sort of thing that is best read at the bottom of the page, in a footnote."[31]

Distance, then, does not necessarily mean estrangement, split-offness, or isolation. Distance (made by separating fused elements) may provide space in which to perceive and receive self and other, or in the instance of poison ivy, of physical vulnerability and threatening oil. Such distance is space-making and the antidote to being overwhelmed, whether we are talking about hypersensitivity and toxic plant, parent and child, or the mystic and God.

The philosopher-theologian Jean-Luc Marion maintains that Christ's ascension bestowed the necessary distance on his disciples and all subsequent followers. The intervening space allows believers to perceive that Christ is no longer localized—identified with one place and historical time, and accessible only to people in that space and time—but lives everywhere for all time, and hence is available to everyone. His physical bodily nearness gives way to his all-encompassing spiritual presence through his ascending distance, which allows everyone else enough space to receive his presence.[32]

Eastern and Homeopathic Perspectives

From the point of view of Chinese medicine, the super-allergic person's overreaction amounts to too much *yang* element—meaning hot, driving energy—in the case of poison ivy, it is a sort of fire on the skin.[33] Itching and scratching inflames the skin and makes it burn, as if fire had ignited it. [34] This overreaction takes us too far from the center, at too great a "distance from equilibrium."[35] In contrast to the alchemical operation, where some measure of distance must be established (a kind of separation into opposites that can then properly conjoin), here a different healing operation must be installed. Neither too little nor too great a distance must be instituted. Distance here means too far-removed from "stillness," that still-point of all movements where Dōgen locates the self. The right balance is needed between opposite extremes, the just proportion of yang (fiery, active energy) and *yin* (receptive, cool, moist, calm energy). In this symbolic vocabulary, eruptions of poison ivy occur due to an excess of pulsating, driving, active, fiery energy that puts us at too great a distance from the center. Dean Black, writing on allergies, notes the similar perceptions of the Nobel-prize scientist Ilya Prigogine that "shows such a striking parallel between the ancient Chinese ideas and modern science" that:

> Order appears to be a compromise between two antagonists: the nonlinear chemical-like process—and the transport-like process. . . . Disturbing the delicate balance between these two competing actors leads to such qualitative changes as an erratic state in which each element of the system acts on its own; or, on the contrary a "homeostatic" or fossillike state. . . . Complexity, therefore, appears to be limited on opposite sides by [two] different kinds of disorder.[36]

Homeopathy recognizes the same problem of imbalance between extremes (yin and yang) in psychosomatic conditions.

The "whole host of allergic conditions affecting skin" can be traced to "disturbed protective organization and stabilizing equilibrium" related to the energy fields of the remedies *calcarea* and *magnesia*.[37] The substances share in common some positive and negative properties: "Mentally and on the personality level, the tendency of walling off an inner stabilization means a leaning towards separateness and self-finding. While in its favorable aspect this means independence, in its less favorable, one-sided exaggeration it is withdrawal from people, tendency to go it alone, loss of social contact, stubbornness and obstinacy."[38] Self-finding means the absence of dependency because it is unmet. We try to rely, instead, on holding ourselves up.

Looking for the individual characteristics of these two substances leads the homeopathist to look for the image or guiding symbol that best expresses their force-pattern. For *calcarea*, it is found in chalk and the oyster-shell; for *magnesia*, it is found in the greenness of the plant, and the lightning-like explosive effect of magnesium in flash bulbs or incendiary bombs.[39] In the image of chalk we find the yin pole, of "passivity, immobility, standstill"; and in the image of the greenness of plants the yang pole of the renewing energy of life standing in contrast to its destruction by too much explosive energy.[40]

Insofar as these remedies might be used symbolically to understand the rhythmic flow of contraction and expansion of opposite energy patterns in the skin, we can see that those who suffer from the ivy disease are caught in a collision of opposing tendencies. The Ivy Leaguers are stuck at once in both immobile passivity, trying to restrain action and movement so as not to set off convulsive itching, and also in the besieged skin expressing explosive activity, destructive change, and aggressive irritation.[41] On the one hand, as if in an extreme of *calcarea*, sufferers may be too permeable to the influences of their surroundings, too easily affected, hypersensitive, as certainly poison ivy allergic people are. They become infected even from the air; the disease builds a thick armor of blisters; they are confined to the isolation of bed, unable to go about freely with others or touch anyone. On the other hand, as if in an extreme of *magnesia*, the impulsive, undisciplined, violent capacity is manifested on the skin, which erupts, bursts, weeps, and convulses in spasms of painful itching, like a storm not finding any other outlet, except to play itself out on the body.[42]

Genetic Influence?

One other physical fact may apply here, though the genetic influence has proved difficult to verify. In an era when age 36 was considered the dangerous end of a woman's birth-giving capacity, my mother endured an arduous pregnancy coming to term with me, her third child. Because of her low blood-sugar, her doctor advised her to eat candy during her pregnancy. She weighed over 200 pounds when it came time for her to deliver. Before any of her pregnancies, she weighed 115 pounds; after the birth of my brother and sister, she weighed about 135. In delivering me, she went past her delivery date for some weeks, worrying her friends and family so much that her beloved brother-in-law, who was singing in *Aida* at the Metropolitan Opera, phoned to tell her that in the second act, in the triumphal entry scene, Lily Pons would sustain a high A for thirty seconds and when my mother heard that note on the radio she was "to bear down and get rid of that baby!" She did, and was taken to the hospital with initial contractions. But they petered out.

Finally, her doctor elected to administer a drug to induce labor, but that simply aroused an intense adverse reaction. It made her itch! She swelled up to even greater size, so big she was unable to lie down on the gurney conducting her to the delivery room, but arrived, instead, sitting up like a big balloon. The itching was convulsive, violent, unceasing, plaguing, horrible. The nurses had to tie her hands to prevent her gouging at her flesh. Was there then a cellular transmission to the baby of this intense irritation, this allergic propensity that produces paroxysms of scratching? Was I in some intra-womb communication induced into sensitivity to allergic responses that manifest in itching? No other allergies beset me until mild hay-fever varieties in my 40s.

In concert with the stance of Chinese and homeopathic medicine that examines the constellation of events, both attitudinal and factual, psychological and physical, in which a malady arises, my mother was far from her center, before, during, and after this third birth. Before her delivery, she suffered acute physical discomfort, enough to worry people about her survival, and enough for her doctor to tell her that she was to risk no more pregnancies. This prohibition struck her like a blow. She wanted more children. During labor and at the actual birth, the labor-inducing drug produced a violent allergic response in her, making her miserable, completely overcome by virulent itching and scratching. Her baby—me—was 10 pounds, swimming in quarts of amniotic fluid which rushed over the delivery table to the floor, and so overdue that I was clothed in a caul and had grown long hair and long fingernails. And I was a she. My mother wished for four boys. She got only one, along with two girls, this last one putting paid to any more children. All these factors did not make for a happy, centered, joyful celebration, but rather one suffused with sorrow.

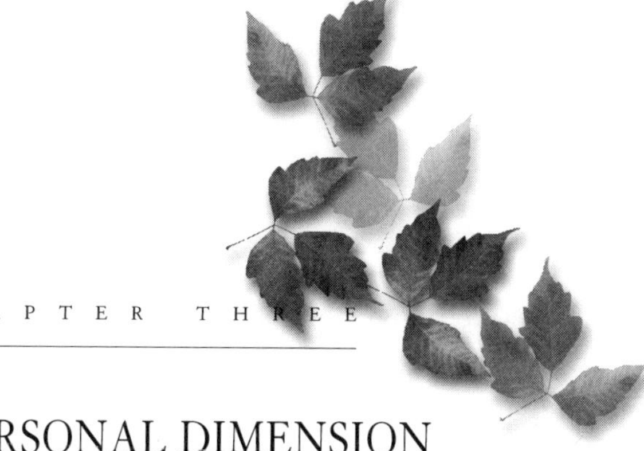

CHAPTER THREE

THE PERSONAL DIMENSION

The needful thing is not to know *the truth but to* experience *it. Not to have an intellectual conception of things, but to find our way to the inner, and perhaps wordless, irrational experience. . . . Nothing is more important than finding the way to these far-off goals.*[1]

THE QUESTION FROM MY ANALYSAND, ABOUT WHAT meaning there could be in the fact that every year I contracted poison ivy, initiated a deep shift in my perceptions. The question acted as a door into another perspective. The future possibility of receiving a communication—that this besetting repetitive nuisance might hold unguessed value—opened up a large part of my past. I began to ask, as if a reporter, about the who, what, when, where, and why of my ivy affliction, looking for its cause in my past: Jung's analytical-reductive method. I looked for a purpose this repetitious allergy was tending toward in the future: Jung's synthetic-prospective method. What broke into me then was a clustering of simultaneous, coinciding, opposite events and attitudes—of my own body and mind and those of people around me in the past, of past sufferings with poison ivy in my body, and future sufferings in my psyche, of conscious thoughts about the purpose of this vexing allergic reaction, and unconscious unveilings through symptom and dream of meaning already there awaiting my meeting it while I was also creating it: Jung's notion of synchronicity now operating as a method of inquiry and disclosure.

The upshot of this riotous clustering of opposites seemingly from all sides at once, this cacophony, was insight into psychological method. We cannot go back into past "object-relations" except as the future discloses their ongoing unfurling life in us now. What Jung calls the final cause uncovers the original cause. The purpose toward which we tend sheds light on factors that first prompted attitudes and actions. What we are making of past experiences now is much like Loewald's idea of the present ego reorganizing the past by re-viewing it, or like Augustine's *memoria*, where the past is not dead information, inert and finished, but alive in relation to us now.[2] The past becomes available only as the future opens up. Only with what Bion calls *A Memoir of the Future* do we gain access to the past.[3]

The analytic-reductive method that Jung describes as resolving a present dream or symptom "into its memory components and the underlying instinctual processes" which lead us to "memory-complexes that refer to external situations," breaks down when the "symbols can no longer be reduced to personal reminiscences or aspirations, that is, when the images of the collective unconscious begin to appear."[4] We exhaust our personal memory, which is about finite events and persons, and is itself finite. Interpreting only with reference to "objects" external to ourselves—mother, father, sibling, child—also comes to an end because our fellow creatures bare their finitude, showing us that they do not possess the great power with which we endow them. Thus reducing our present symptom down to its origin in the past and to the people whose invasion or neglect of us "caused" our symptoms, eventually brings causality to an end.

The reduction leads to an archetypal dimension that presents us with another point of view. To deny this, or fail to see it, leads us into inflation or deflation because the archetypal energies then can express themselves only through personal material rather than being seen as a distinct kind of energy in themselves. Archetypal energies then invade and inflate personal memories and affects. The torrent of affect that expresses itself in a dream, for example, reaches us as a huge downpour that so saturates the ground that the excess can only be run off down gullies into the earth below, down rivers back to the sea. Such an image cannot be expressed through personal symbols alone, say of a woman, the dreamer, crying. The dream is showing her, instead, that the waters of sorrow well exceed personal tears. They flood the ground, they overflow even the earth's containers and must run back into the deep underground, back to the ocean. If the dreamer tries to live this torrent only as personal feelings, she will either be drowned in sorrow (which is a kind of deflation), or she will inflate her personal sadness to archetypal proportions. She might, for example, assume the grandiose role of a *mater dolorosa*, who, like the mother of God, weeps for the sins of the world. The symbol of the torrent is too large for individual terms and must be conjugated as part of the whole human family's symbolic grammar. I could say that the reiterated poison ivy outbreaks (as with anyone's automatically recurring symptoms) was due precisely to the big camel of archetypal energy trying to pass through the too small needle's-eye of my allergy complaint.

Only now, more than a decade later, do I see that then, when the question of the significance of poison ivy so stunned me, a shift of monumental proportions, from present to future, was inaugurated. I did not only ask where this pestiferous bother came from, but also, now, where it was tending. To what end did this ridiculous childhood plague keep repeating itself? For who at the age of 50 was still being annoyed as if they were 5, or at most 15, with gooey, itchy, outbreaks? Instead of simply feeling humiliated, my curiosity quickened. What was the message here, so patiently repeated, deemed important enough to go on being recounted every year? And if it was important, to whom was it so? My body? Some reality speaking through my body to my spirit?

These questions partake of Jung's synthetic-prospective method that amplifies the bits of memory-complexes uncovered by reductive analysis "with all conscious means at our disposal" while detaching them "from their external causes," seeing them "as tendencies or components of the subject, and reunites them with that subject."[5] Thus what I had seen as restated ordeals, as "distortions" of normal growth and health, I now began to see as archetypal affects and impulses of the unconscious, symbolizing its collective layers, pressing to get through to consciousness to be seen in their "own" right. I shifted from despair over still not conquering this stubborn foe to wonder at my own persistent blindness and deafness. I was not receiving the message that was repeatedly being sent to me. I shifted from ego attitudes of enduring, evading, and curing poison ivy to a determined inquiry. What meaning was being displayed? What was functioning in me as a living thing?

This living thing existed in my body, not in my mind or emotions. The irony, the real humor of the situation, emerged full force when I asked the body what it had to say through poison ivy. Once asked, the body all but bowed out. Like a faithful dog from another kingdom, once its message was accepted, the dog went home. I began to dream of poison ivy attacks instead. No more poison ivy attacks occurred.[6] The body's affliction was rescued into image instead.

These conjunctions of body-mind and instinct-spirit ushered me into a different place, not just a different perspective or attitude. Skin is a way of meeting the world; it is the surface where inner meets outer. I was shifted into a psychoid space, where mind and body each had its own consciousness. Matter and psyche bore me forward toward any meaning I could find or construct. Even in the writing of this manuscript, my body still plays such a role. It itches, or produces tiny little blisters; it brings me low, feeling sickish, somehow invalid. It escorts me into a different field where all the parts converge, clash, compete, and finally converse with each other to make up a bigger picture closer to a whole. The direction of the prospective view gives way to a surrounding synchronistic view of this childhood symptom.[7]

Using the analytical-reductive method, we look at the symptom, here poison ivy episodes, from an ego point of view. We uncover what we defend against and why we do so. Using the synthetic-prospective method, we look at the poison ivy attacks from a Self point of view, to discover what it is trying to assemble through the distress, what this distress symbolizes. We open, in sum, to what the Self is engineering. Using a method based on synchronicity, we see that both previous methods clashed and resounded through each other. The cause that the ego uncovers now acts as the occasion for the Self to generate meaning and show pattern.

But we must understand that meaning and pattern do not fall upon us ready-made. Without the ego pushing and pulling—like shoving a broken bone in place, bringing focus and dissolving all focus, both concentrating and dispersing any order we would impose on the unconscious—meaning does not unfold. When it finally does so, it seems to arrive as if from beyond our efforts, but our efforts are in fact essential; they go out to meet it, to wait a hundred years for it if necessary, to hack through a hedge to get it, to dig it up, to eat it, to make a vessel for it.

The distortion through violent eruptions of the skin in the infestation of poison ivy now displays itself as a new beginning, a nascent symbol that can integrate conflicting emotions, join inner experience to outer people, a fledgling self to the world around it. What I discovered, and labeled as a dissociation in this life-long plague of poison ivy, turned out to be the beginning of differentiation. What I first analyzed in cause and effect terms as stemming from what had originated in my past, revealed itself now as going far beyond any cause. My body exceeded the container of causality. It was as if causality was being used as an occasion for the body to speak about something else. Like the painter Paul Klee, who saw that the "principle of repetition" means that "any number of the parts can be added or taken away without changing the rhythmic character," I now saw the whole attack from another side.[8] It was not simply a repetitious cause-and-effect procedure, but a recurrent movement as well, a rhythmic process, a form full of beat, a swinging, singing out of meaning. What I had seen as blocked communication and hence irksome compulsive repetition, I now saw as an effort toward a ritual-in-the-making, to communicate through the symbols of body-speech and the skin envelope, not only feeling, but something much larger. The skin disease was trying to create a new ground in which the consubstantiation of meaning and matter could grow, where objective reality could become subjective human experience.

Jung links such moments to religious experience. He writes, "So long as the collective unconscious and the individual psyche are coupled together without being differentiated, no progress can be made . . . the boundary cannot be crossed. . . . But the [archetypal] energy becomes serviceable again by being brought into play through man's [sic] conscious attitude toward the collective unconscious. The religions have established this cycle of energy in a concrete way by means of ritual communion with the gods."[9] These are moments "when the gods intervene," occasions which bring into focus an attitude of "'*Religio*' in the sense of a 'careful consideration' of unknown dangers and agencies. . . ."[10] But who knows what we will encounter—a demon or a god? Certainly a vicious attack of ivy suggests the former. Jung advises: "if we must take the plunge, we need a good deal of 'trust in God' or 'faith'. . . . Thus unsought and unsuspected, the question creeps in of one's religious attitude to fate."[11]

Investigating the memories of poison ivy demanded such a trust from me. The shift in perception engendered a willingness to give up needing to know where this would lead. It was like setting out on a sea voyage with no land ahead. Though Jung describes this kind of an adventure as moving into a "mode of apprehension mediated by the archetypes and capable of uniting the opposites," for the person undertaking the voyage this means nothing more than being tossed about by great waves.[12] And, indeed, opening to my memories of poison ivy amounted to huge invasions of affect—mainly of weeping in unnamable sorrow, languishing in unspeakable silence, fearing undefinable danger in the sense of being undefended against falling into nothingness. This was really a departure from all the ego-needs for safe space.

This whole poison ivy part of my life was not repressed, but dissociated, separate, encapsulated. But it did exist. I could mention it, remember it, get at it, but I never brought it up and no one ever asked about it. With my patient's query about its meaning, and my open consent to the question, this whole cargo of living heaved up into the near distance. All my senses galvanized to apprehend it: I could hear the death-like silence that had sealed this part of my life into a separate chamber; I caught a glimpse of the surface shininess of the large tight blisters and smelled the liquid oozing from sores; I could feel the horny, tough texture of heels, knees, elbows, even ears, hardened from layers of infection. Memory elicited everything, even tastes. No food or liquid satisfied when it had to make its way past swollen lips and painful gums.

The Skin

In taking a psychosomatic perspective, the body part selected to speak for the psyche's experience proves crucial. Here the largest of body organs, the skin, plays the dominant role, itself a container, boundary, and communicator. Skin is vital. Without the greater part of it remaining intact, we cannot survive. Damage to skin brings the threat of annihilation. Skin forms the frontier for relationship between "I" and neighbor, a point of contact and of differentiation. Skin creates the limiting membrane that allows us to cohere into a unit, and establishes a boundary, marking "me" off from "not-me," self from world. It contains our inner life and differentiates us from others.

Skin is the basis of contact with the world and others. It is a medium of exchange, conjugated in all the senses. It must be touched. When it is, it moves us emotionally to pleasure, to comfort, to security, to pain and terror, even to rage if invaded. Skin can be sniffed and it, itself, can smell. We look at skin, and behold it in a beautiful newborn, or in a lover. One man, for example, seeking analysis in the wake of the break-up of a relationship with the woman he had felt most deeply about in his whole life spoke movingly of her skin and any woman's skin. The scent of it, its softness, its lambent texture evoked in him the desire to be enveloped by it, next to it, touching it, touched by it. I could hear a child held securely in his mother's arms, a man in ecstatic embrace with his beloved, and still something more—as if skin itself bore to him the scent, the taste and touch, the holding of the transcendent. To come to the end of this significant relationship, even if appropriate, made him feel exiled from being itself.

Skin can shimmer, glow, or look muddy, absolutely opaque. Its textures change in different parts of the body, with every change of temperature. Goosebumps, chafing, contrast with shimmering softness. We taste skin when we lick it, in lovemaking, or in some Asian practices of medicine. Do we hear skin? Certainly when scratched, its resonances reach our ears, as for example its whispery sigh when stroked, yet it makes no sound when it bleeds. Skin moistens, sweats, or dries out and wrinkles up. We shed our skin daily, hence its symbolic link to the serpent, to the toad. Underneath the old cracked skin emerges a new young body-covering. A former analysand in her 50s, who returned for a few sessions after suffering a life-threatening illness, showed baby-fresh unlined skin, an unguessed benefit from the ravaging side-effects of chemotherapy for the treatment of cancer. The old skin had dried up, turned brown from the drugs, and peeled away; she said, "This new young skin was my reward."

Skin localizes us, makes a space in time for an "I" to dwell in the body. Skin is the organ of incarnation. Without it, we do not coagulate into a definite form of existing. We inhabit no residence, possess no container in which to dwell, no site from which to interact with others. We speak of being at home in our skins; of having a skin of our own, yet it also puts our psyche in contact with the external world. Disorders of the skin bespeak trouble, not feeling safely enclosed in definite form, nor open at the same time to contact with others, to the whole world. Our inside and outside commerce suffers.

Psychoanalysts speak wisely about the skin as a psychosomatic zone of combat: "such suspended ideas can express themselves easily . . . in certain skin troubles for instance. . . . The idea is like an autonomous being that wants a body so much that it even incarnates itself . . . it comes down into reality like the runes which were hatched out by Odin when he was hanging on the tree."[13] The selection of body-organ depends on "the one at which the existence of a person happens to be carried out at the time. . . . The somatic phenomena which push themselves into the limelight . . . belong exclusively to the world-relation at which a human being is existing at the time, though only in a dammed-up way."[14] If skin is the selected organ, it always "involves ego distress. . . . The basis of psycho-somatics is live anatomy. . . . The tissues are alive and they are part of a whole animal, and are affected by the varying psychic states of that animal."[15] Of all the psychosomatic disorders, allergy is the most difficult to place, and poison ivy above all, because it is *not* thought to be psychosomatic in its origins at all, but simply the effect of contact with its cause—exposure to an oily vine. Nonetheless, I locate poison ivy within psychosomatic phenomena, at the very least because the psyche can load dissociated emotional experiences onto poison ivy outbreaks.

A psychosomatic disorder dissociates psyche and soma. It splits the person from what Winnicott calls the environmental provision, apportioning the body to one set of doctors and the psyche to another.[16] Khan writes of using our symptoms as a way of "'corseting' . . . unintegrated states, instead of tolerating that inevitable nonbeing which is inherent to personalized living in one's skin."[17] We need what Anzieu calls "*le moi-peau*," the me-skin, that serves as a precursor to the ego and its attributes. Before a formed ego exists, we can "enact the parent's predicament on our own 'le moi-peau.'"[18] Anzieu asks the intriguing question, "what if thought were as much an affair of the skin as of the brain?"[19] Nina Coltart recognizes the "dense and enigmatic code" of a psychosomatic symptom, saying we must "ask what is the unthinkable content slouching along" in its "darkness." She asks further, "How do we build a bridge which really *holds* over the secret area of the body-mind divide? Can the unthinkable become thinkable?"[20] We must also ask, as does Bollas, to whom is the symptom addressed and for what purpose? What communication to the environment is being uttered? To attract attention? To be a nuisance?[21]

In the system of chakras of Hindu psychology, the skin is the sense organ associated with the heart region, the chakra of feeling for oneself and, beyond self, for others. This heart realm is manifested in Shiva who here wears a golden tiger skin and has blue skin, symbolizing nonattachment to worldly pleasures, honors, and humiliations, and flowing with a purifying stream of self-knowledge. This knowledge consists in knowing that *I* am *That*, manifesting in air as energy to the entire body. At this heart center of energy, the practice of Kundalini Yoga aims to attain a balance of masculine and feminine energies through meditation on the perception of divine grace in all existence.[22]

At the heart chakra level (*Anahata*), the bounteousness of our energy to expand toward accepting and embracing our self depends on securing our existence at the first root chakra (*Muladhara*), where issues of survival are paramount. With specific reference to the organ of the skin at this foundation level of existence, the central question is: Do we live in a grounded, intact container? If not, fear plagues us; we feel shaky, overly stressing the nervous system and adrenal glands, pervaded by anxiousness over whether we can remain in being.[23] Our sense of aliveness and well-being depends on a feeling of support *by* and rootedness *in* the mysterious central source of the ground beneath us. This kind of rooting provides stability, which we feel as a taken-for-granted right to exist, to be here. Being grounded expresses itself in our sense of holding our boundaries, having our own rooted lives, and even sealing our container for the work of inward transformation. Roots grow down within us and out beyond us to be nourished by parents, caretakers, the world around us.[24] This root chakra represents our connection to the tribal group into which we are born. Energetically, the power and issues of tribal containment (or its lack) relate to the health of our immune system.[25] Disruption of the skin, which poison ivy visits on its sufferers, as well as being an immune disorder, aggravates the deficiency of these strong roots and also expresses the fear that our dependency on others will not be met. We do not feel part of the tribe, but rather as if outside looking in. While we endorse the unified beliefs of the group, the tribal belief system, we also feel alienated from the group.

At the fourth chakra level of the heart, the lack of a secure rooted foundation at the first chakra level shows up as the demon of grief. Great sorrow pervades the heart. The self has not been held and beheld. Mending occurs as we listen to "the body's subtle communications . . . allowing the mind to behold our experience in the body." In addition, at this heart-chakra level, we fear we are unable to protect ourselves emotionally.[26]

The task at this heart-chakra level is to love and be loved, to become "unstuck," by embracing what is, both within us and in others. Loving ourselves means contacting the "wounded child" within us who still suffers under emotional patterns of painful memories, negative self-images, and fearful attitudes. If we are to become unstuck, we must unseat the authority of these hurtful presuppositions.[27] In this fourth region, we move beyond ourselves to promote relationships with others and with life itself: "In beholding the self, we witness a miraculous manifestation of divine energy living right inside us, with all its hopes and fears, joys and tears. This witnessing is 'the heart of the heart.' It brings us to the sacred."[28] And, according to Myss, this healing energy can build only within a securely contained body. She goes on to say that when the skin container is broken and ravaged, "grief sits on the chakra like a stone. When our heart is heavy with grief, it is hard to open, it is even hard to breathe. . . . We may feel dead inside."[29]

The highest, seventh chakra level (*Sahasrara*) connects us to our spiritual nature and allows it to guide our daily physical and psychological lives. Its energy seeks to align to the eternal Divine in the here and now. At the physical level the nodal point is the top of the head but, for our purposes here, it is important to note that "the energy of the seventh chakra influences that of the major body systems: the central nervous system, the muscular system, and the *skin*."[30] Thus the poison ivy syndrome registers distress at the basic level of survival, the heart level of love, and the highest spiritual level of contact with the divine. On all three levels distress is expressed as disorder of the skin.

What, then, in the poison ivy scenario, is the idea that seeks expression? In Jung's words, what is the secret rune that reveals itself out of sacrifice, like Odin's when hanging on a tree? What is the dammed-up area of relation to existence, as Boss describes it? What animal is at risk, in Winnicott's words, and what function does the gap perform which the symptom enforces between psyche and soma? Why can't the poison ivy victim tolerate non-being, but instead needs what Khan calls "corseting" to hold together? What, as Bollas asks, is the parent's predicament that the poison ivy child enacts on her skin? What is the skin thinking, to use Anzieu's words?

Can we crack the poison ivy code, as Coltart puts it, and put into words the unthinkable anxiety it portrays through the skin? What survival is at risk at the root-chakra level, and what is the wound to the heart chakra that this skin affliction seeks to express? What divine energy at the spirit-chakra level is blocked from incarnating that would relieve the skin distress? In Joyce McDougall's words,[31] what is the bio-logic that seeks to become psycho-logic in the poison ivy symptom?

Many opposites collide in poison ivy suffering. In between the opposites a liminal space slowly constructs itself. The body collects, expresses, and knits together conflicting tensions. Any symptom attempts to communicate and defend. But frequently, in the schools of depth psychology, we use the concept of defense in a pejorative fashion. Pointing out a defense as a defense too often makes us feel defensive, as if we were doing something wrong. Defenses aim to protect, to offer shelter where none exists. But they remain amazing creations, even if neurotic. And they usually work. People survive because of them, even if at psychic or physical cost. To pay a bill is better than to die.

The Gap Between Opposites

The opposites that collect around poison ivy are many, and involve me, my family, and go beyond my family to what we might call the human family and to its afflictions. The skin itself, when healthy, harnesses both permeability and impermeability, elasticity and desiccation, conserving and shedding, inner vulnerability and outer protection, both narcissistic and sexual satisfaction.[32] The skin itself operates as a liminal transitional state, somewhere between psyche and body and world.

A first set of opposites in a poison ivy attack startles the observer: "Don't Touch!" conflicts with "Help me! Hold me!" A severe outbreak of poison ivy creates a body-armor of hard, tight, small, unyielding blisters that grow up from under the skin in four or five layers, making a dense shield that cannot be penetrated. For example, on my wrists or ankles, these tight, tiny blisters formed chains, like a suit of mail, that prevented any bending, as if I wore iron gloves and shin guards. On the skin's surface, the blisters grew larger still, pressured by fluid about to burst out of them, making me hypersensitive to any contact, however light. Such body-armor prevents any touching or holding; suggesting, instead, a person become stiff with self-holding, a self-holding gone rigid. I could not bend hands or feet, elbows or knees. This protective covering enforced rigid posture, marking off precise limits by thickening the membrane between inner and outer, me and not-me. The suffering skin crusts over with blisters broken and reformed: it is jagged, crumbly. The flaking skin shouts: "No Trespassing! Keep Off!" The pain that this isolation brings is defended by a condensed viscid armor. The defense is not inarticulate: on the opposite side, this skin is also weeping, endlessly weeping, crying out for help and a soothing touch. I was surprised to remember that I had never cried when I had poison ivy. I see now that my skin did it for me; it never stopped crying. Maybe, in Anzieu's words, that was the thought the skin was thinking—a breakdown in the task of self-holding. The despair of never being held, and the strain of prematurely holding myself up, broke through my skin, if not my words.

The skin wept fluid, serum, blood. Even healing did not stop the weeping. The soppiness of poison ivy commands steady, repeated care throughout the day, and at least once during the night. One has to mop up the tears, so to speak. Changing bandages, putting clean gauze strips on the most oozing sores, applying either alcohol or some astringent to cauterize the dripping blisters—all this physical weeping calls for care from others. Curiously, I have no memory of who did this, though I think it must have been my mother. My second mother, the cook, did not do it, nor did my father, even though he was a medical doctor. I did not see my brother or sister, nor the cook's husband, my great pal with whom I had gone fishing and caught the infection, instead of a fish. On the leafy banks of the canal, I must have stood, sat, or lay down on a blanket in the midst of the dread ivy for the whole afternoon.

My body communicated my weeping to my mother as an argument for holding and being held, but at a proper distance. And it called the best out of her, which was very good indeed. Skilled as a nurse before her marriage, she excelled in such care. Neither intrusive nor sentimental, she communicated care through fresh, cool bed-linen, a softly shadowed room to spare my eyes and lessen the heat, tiny snacks of cracked ice for my swollen mouth and gums, or a sip of Coke through a glass straw that was bent so a neck rigid with blisters could reach it. Sometimes little vases with a few bright flowers brightened the table next to a bed festooned with medicine bottles—the familiar pink calamine, a dark brown alcoholic "Ivy Dry," and a new bright mustard-yellow liquid we were trying out, which sadly proved no good.

In the space between the body-armor repudiating all contact, on one hand, and my wordless crying out for solace and holding, on the other, the poison ivy body created appropriate caring—neither too close, nor too far away. Poison ivy set the proper distance. I do not remember any conversation about the affliction. My mother, in her nurse persona, was a matter-of-fact, sensate, down-to-earth person with a witty sense of humor. Her robust attitude, if it did not get too hearty and cheery, gave me confidence I would get well again. You just did what poison ivy cures necessitated, and did not mope. This attitude was not sufficient as my yearly repetition of poison ivy indicated, though none of the subsequent attacks reached the pitch of the crisis when I was 10. After that grave incident, I remember caring for myself, much in the manner my mother had cared for me—doing the chores of washing, bandaging, applying gauze strips and lotion, not fretting, just getting through it. Perhaps my attacks were repeated because too little sharing of feeling occurred between my mother and me directly, but only indirectly, myself speaking through my encrusted body and she through her nursing. We acted out what the disease communicated in its own terms, about not enough real holding during the rest of the year. But the body did speak its own dialect, and we managed in the space between the opposites of, "Do not trespass," and "Please embrace me," to fashion a kind of caring that brought me through. My attacks also expressed faith in my mother's resilience and in her defenses against sorrow. I expressed her sorrow and she mopped it up.

What looms from these affect-laden memories is an unmet dependency as the "normal" state of affairs that bred in me, prematurely, a capacity to regard my parents (both sets of them) as distinct and separate objects[33] instead of gradually emerging from dependence on them. My imagining is that my birth coincided with sorrow in my mother for the physical stress she suffered (which included violent itching!) and especially for the ending of her child-bearing. Around that time, too, I believe, a change that lasted a number of years occurred in her marriage, associated with greater emotional frustration and less physical intimacy with my father. Typologically, my mother and I were opposites; she an extrovert, and, though brilliant, also blunt, bursting with undigested thoughts; I an introvert, hidden, not finding easy expression for feelings and intuitions that ran deep. Her brute logic met up with my fledgling efforts to speak the nonrational, felt sense of meaning. She told me that as a child, I did not let her hold me, and there is a photo that shows me pulling away rather than yielding to her arms. Something in the air between us produced an allergy, a hesitancy, a hypersensitivity and a guardedness. My mother said she never knew what I was thinking. I felt she never waited to ask.

My Slavic parents, the cook and the houseman, were of the earth, peasants from Yugoslavia, without even a last name when they emigrated to this country. The officials left the space for their name blank because they could not tell what it was. Ever afterward they went by the last name of Mr. and Mrs. Blank. She was illiterate, a genius at cooking, given to harsh shaming of her charges, with a big laugh, durable and tough. He, barely literate (spelling phonetically, so that I had to read aloud his letters to me from the war to sound out the words), was softer, unable, as his wife was, though for different reasons, to behead the chickens with a kitchen knife. He wept while she struck boldly. He liked to sing, and joke, and work hard.

My father, who loved his work as a surgeon, provided a steady background presence, but his loving felt distant, for he always left early in the morning to perform surgery, and returned late for dinner at night. An equable, warm, calm feeling emanated from him, but he had no immediate presence. All four of my parents gave me a great deal of freedom, or just simply left me on my own. I would be gone for whole afternoons, roaming the countryside with the dogs, though it was my cat who held me in being. No one asked where I went for so long, so often, nor where I had been when I returned. I enjoyed, and endured, a great deal of solitude as a child.

Winnicott links being physically held with attaining an indwelling of psyche in soma. Clearly some holes occurred in me, which I displayed each year through broken skin. I developed self-holding early on, and poison ivy attacks were communiqués that I wanted to be held—in attention, in body, in love. The psyche made use of an allergy to poison ivy to break down the effort of self-maintenance, to break up the defense of isolating true feelings, to break through self-holding to appeal to others for support.[34]

Premature self-holding bequeaths us early perception of the limits of the holding of us by others, by life itself. For behind my own small issues loomed a vision of nothing being there, an endless gap in being, and an accompanying affective despair. A distinct memory from age 8 is of seeing and feeling the shock that there easily could be nothing instead of something. Sheer absence of anything in contrast to everything existing around me joined up with this perception of limits—my parents' limits, the limits to their happiness, the limits of language, the limits of the rootedness of my second parents, a persistent note of lack and hopelessness beneath our whole family's lovely life in a big house, in a beautiful country, with plenty to eat, and all sorts of luxuries. I felt the force of nothingness, of abyss and void, the danger of annihilation through the gaps in the meetings of my own dependency; and through those gaps, the nothingness, the nonbeing that can annihilate any of us at any time. In the horrendous late 20th-century plight of Yugoslavian refugees fleeing first from the armed conflict in Croatia and Bosnia, and then later in Kosovo, I felt disturbed on a deep preconscious level, as well as consciously distressed like everyone else. Here again was annihilation writ large, as a people lost in a moment or in a few weeks, not only their homes and possessions, but also their identity papers, their country, their health, their families. At any moment our existence could be torn up, torn through, thrown away.

Poison ivy offered a good focus for the impact of this metaphysical attitude on my immediate life as a child. I caught it each year, partly because of exposure to an emotional attitude of benign neglect, as well as to the ubiquitous plant. No warnings sounded to circumscribe my daily outdoor wanderings, to indicate places to avoid the baneful oak, sumac, or ivy. The river and its canal boasted the reputation of lush greenness, but no prohibition stopped me going fishing there with the houseman. No instruction was enforced to make me memorize the enemy—to identify it, to avoid the stems, leaflets, colors, vines, and berries of the infectious plants. None of us took any notice.

More striking still, no recourse was taken to the medical armament necessary to heal the infection when it struck me so severely at age 10. An analysand of mine who came for treatment from the south, with its own lush greenness, one day recalled her own felling by the noxious ivy, a case so harsh that she was rushed to the hospital. Hospital? My countertransference registered. Was a hospital possible? Was it helpful? My father, as chief of staff, possessed easy access to all facilities, to all sorts of doctors, as provided by the age of specialization. I do not remember him even being in the room where I lay, though mother had brought me down from my third floor rooms to the north guest room during that awful attack. It was more convenient, closer to their room, on the same floor. But treatment drew on nothing stronger than Fels Naptha soap and calamine lotion, though we did try out all the new cream remedies as they appeared, and all, uniformly, proved ineffective.

In that November episode many decades later, when a doctor prescribed prednisone, I was in awe of its power. It worked from the inside, as if sapping the blisters from within, so that in eight days the more egregious lesions quietly reduced to faded marks. When prednisone suppresses the immune system, our body then stops swelling, producing fluids to flush out the enemy that is no longer there. The body stops fighting the presence of Nothing. Such massive defense is no longer needed. We become unarmed, defenseless. Our mute appeal for help conveys itself through our helplessness to protect ourselves. The "danger that cannot be thought about" displays itself in a broken body, a body whose container is torn.[35]

The one attack I suffered, after beginning this present investigation, sprang from the same benign neglect I had experienced as a child.[36] No sadism, at least of a conscious kind, was directed toward me, no move to hurt, or to indulge cruel power. Instead, I fell victim to a laconic refusal to come into focused awareness that this plant could hurt me seriously and protection from it could be gained if we all made the effort to be attentive. As I said earlier, I, too, refused the intercession of consciousness.[37] As with my parents, it was too much trouble for me that summer day to rouse myself to proscribe and prohibit, to go into the house and suit up in my asbestos-like clothes. Nor did I cease from brush-cutting, but instead just discounted the danger from the lurking ivy. I treated myself with the same benign neglect I had experienced as a child. I abandoned taking care of myself. I acted out instead of reflecting on and choosing a means of self-protection when exposed to the danger that my body harbored knowledge of from my early environment. The subsequent three-inch long blisters up and down my inner calves shattered any feigned distance from vulnerability.

But that attack has been the only one since my beginning this inquiry into the meaning of the allergy. I no longer get poison ivy in that virulent way, though the plant still grows all around me as it always has, for it is notoriously difficult to uproot and extinguish. Conscious now of the perils of benign neglect, I respect the plant's power and protect my vulnerability. The defense now is simpler; the psyche no longer need use the allergy to make contact with the encapsulated psychic pain. Consciousness has interceded and I have felt the psychic pain in full awareness. That releases the body from its burden. What I have treated as a psychosomatic symptom can now be reduced to a contact allergy.

Dreams

The night I got infected by picking poison ivy berries that November, and did not yet know I was already infiltrated by their poison, I dreamed a short dream, noteworthy for its abstract symbolism. The dream presented the word "quincunx" and a sense of pushing something five-sided down a circular shaft. I had no associations to this word, except that five added one to four and hence completed a symbol; I also felt a physical sense of trying to put two things together—a circle and a cornered shape. So I looked up "quincunx" and learned that it designates a five pointed rectangle with four corners and a fifth point in the center, as on dice. Of all geometrical forms, the rectangle seems to be the most rational, a shape preferred for immediate use in life.[38] The quinary represents the human after the Fall, as well as the whole material world, plus the center of quintessence. In Moroccan symbols, the repetition of fives guards against evil; in Islamic rites, five emphasizes religious duties, secret knowledge, and daily prayers. The Chinese count five as the most important number, representing the natural rhythm of life, the order of the cosmos. The quincunx presents the "Cosmic Center" in the form of a cross, where the four cardinal directions meet in the core cross-section, the point of joining of heaven and earth.[39] Five also recalls the five wounds of Christ (feet, hands and side), and the five senses of the soul, which are patterned after the body senses, but apprehend what transcends the physical. When, two days later, I awoke on Monday morning to the knowledge I was in trouble with a serious poison ivy attack, the dream made more sense. This symbol was the first comment that I recall the unconscious ever making through a dream about my chronic allergy. I wrote next to the dream that I certainly need connection to the right order and rhythm, and noted how easily I am thrown off because I have no protection: the poison can just get through, like a gas.

Some months later, when I had time to do more research, I discovered that ivy relates directly to the feminine, denoting a force in need of protection. It is, perhaps, also related to the Greek god Dionysus, hence representing an ecstatic feminine power. Skin relates to birth and rebirth. In Egypt, three skins knotted together symbolize the tail of a panther (my childhood totem and perhaps a clue as to what kind of animal, in Winnicott's words, was at risk here). The three strands represent being born, engendering, and coming into form. Together they mean body, soul, and spirit. The pharaohs and priests of ancient Egypt were thought to pass through the skin and thus to rejuvenate themselves, becoming the panther's tail, clothed in the animal's skins. All this symbolism and the reality it represents, exceeded my actual experience with poison ivy, which was mainly negative, but it aroused in me germinating thoughts. Could poison ivy be associated with renewal?

No dreams showed poison ivy explicitly, but only associations to their imagery. But six months later I dreamed of having three eyes, the third in the middle of my forehead, undefended but covered, so that I could not see all that in fact I did see. I thought then of my utter helplessness before something poisonous, meaning the literal plant, and the covered up nothingness in my family environment (under the surface pressing on all my family members), including my second parents, who didn't even know what name to use when they fled their homeland to save their lives. There could be nothing in life—no hope, no holding in being—for anyone. Poison ivy expressed my distress from my exposure to the suffering surrounding me, covered over in each person I loved—two fathers and two mothers, a sister and a brother—in a house so big that we each had space to carry alone the anguish that beset us. But unspoken anxiety filled up the air around us. My poison ivy rituals each year spoke this distress, made it tangible, curable, and mine alone. Everyone else went on as usual, while I, in my body, was trying to rid myself of something that was not technically there—nothingness. For me, this contact allergy was communicating something that could not be denied; it was a jeopardy that threatened all of us, which I suffered directly.

Soon after, I dreamed of the room, the north guest room, which I associated with being sick with poison ivy. And two months later, I dreamed I was a small child and had lost my mother in a hospital. Looking for her, I could not find her. At the end of the dream, I knew she was dead, and I would never find her. That dream vividly brought to mind being unable to move, being arrested, stopped dead by that dreadful poison ivy attack when 10 years old and moved to that bedroom. The psyche was now dreaming what the infection of poison ivy expressed. Like prednisone, the psyche went beneath the blisters of the physical pain, and rescued into dream images the psychic loss the physical affliction enacted.

Not until two years after the November siege as an adult did I actually dream of poison ivy per se. In the dream, my knees and thighs are armored with poison ivy and "I attack the one who betrayed me." In associating to the images, my notes say, I see the ivy onslaught is very bad, layers and layers of blisters, so that the top of my thighs are rusted and hard, and would take months to heal without medicine like prednisone. But I strip it off and uncover new vulnerable pink skin underneath. It peels back like armor. This body-shield expresses my violent suffering as a child. But here I take a more aggressive attitude and do not sit still. I remove the defense of what Khan calls "corseting," and thus unwrap the "me" that lies beneath it, to face myself. I fight back; I will not be encased; I fight against someone who betrayed me. The dream puts into image form the "unthinkable anxiety" and begins to move me from biological to psychological understanding. Hence the dreams bring to consciousness still more opposites—armor and vulnerability, helplessness and attack, infected skin and new skin.

Aggression, Helplessness, Sex

The psyche used the immune system to display the suffering that I was defenseless against. I was taking something invisible into my system that acted like a poison, and of which I could not rid myself. I made visible this invasion with my frantic somatic efforts to purge myself of its noxious effects. The soma—the body—blindly throws forces into the struggle against psychic pain. Though aggression was bodily displayed in encrusted skin, warding off any touch, nonetheless it was aggression at my own expense. Anzieu notes that a scratching skin disorder is one of the archaic forms of aggression turning against one's own body, to which may be attached an erotic pleasure, somehow to try to tame and make acceptable the panic of being in the grip of uncontrollable forces. Mutilations of the skin are attempts to maintain boundaries of the body and the ego.[40] Ziegler, who promotes what he calls "archetypal medicine" that looks into the value pain and illness might impart, gives a clue to the condensed meanings that poison ivy conveys: "itching is the somatic form of a number of erotic, hostile, even spiritual affects occurring."[41]

Anger, even rage, shows the other side of sorrow in the face of unmet dependency. Venomous poison ivy certainly expresses rage. It is disgusting to look at. All the medications smell. It hurts—one inflicts pain when one scratches. The skin shows angry welts and stubborn sores that refuse to heal swiftly. The affliction gobbles up enormous amounts of time from the one suffering it. I don't remember any fun during these attacks—no games played while confined to bed, no stories told, no books read, no music heard, no drawings made, no company. Psychodynamically, such an assault against the skin can be seen as an attack against the container and hence the containing parents it symbolizes, while at the same time it offers, under the envelope of suffering, some means of restoration of the skin's containing function. Anzieu quotes Pomey-Rey's "safest hypothesis": "The extent of the damage to the skin is proportionate to the depth of psychical harm done."[42] The Greek myth of Marsyas, in one of its versions, shows the hero punished, when his flute playing is judged superior to Apollo's, by being hanged from a tree and flayed. Thus aggression by oneself against oneself is not the only danger. To express aggression outward, toward the other, risks lethal retaliation, as the Marsyas myth shows.

This battle of opposites—aggression both hurled out and held in—is enacted in the poison ivy allergy. Exposed to the outer stimulant (the plant), the oil transgresses the usual boundaries by seeping into other parts of the body that are not yet exposed to the plant. Once the poison is admitted, like a saboteur, it travels secretly throughout our physical system. That is bad enough. To howl with protest and express rage directly for export mounts an even greater threat. Not only might we be dropped forever, and not just by benign neglect, but an atmosphere of annihilation (seen and covered up as the third eye was in my dream) may rise up in response to our protest. It may vanquish us completely instead of being acted out only in the body's repetition compulsion. My poison ivy simultaneously expressed multiple affects: a dead spot of despair; outrage against myself as well as my mother; anxiety about individual identity and about the nonbeing in life itself, and protection of my very right to exist.[43]

Physical pain can bring relief from mental suffering. Primitive longing for closeness, touch, and being held can also admit the precursors of erotic yearnings. Here a primitive erotic crescendo, opposing aggression while fulfilling it, often occurs in the treating of ivy, oak, or sumac incursions. Oak and sumac do what ivy does, only more so, with more stinging pain mixed with the itching. The frenzied incitement to scratch presents real danger; it can push us over into gouging. Most sufferers find relief in the bath. Water soothes the pain, dissolves some of the crusting of the skin, and holds the body in a gentle surrounding. On a symbolic level, is this a return to the fluid of the womb?

The bath, an ever-flowing fountain in alchemical symbolism, expresses an endless source of renewal as well as a flow of interest to the unconscious, what Jung calls "a constant attention, '*religio*' . . . devotion."[44] To submit to this dissolution is to let go of control of the great complexity and tense oppositions expressed in the skin-dialect of poison ivy. To descend into the bath is to yield to a power that transcends these oppositions, for "the water dissolves all created things and leads to the most durable of all products, the mysterious *lapis*."[45] A germinal thought emerges here, that the poison ivy allergy might be serving some transcendent purpose as well as eloquently communicating the meaning of present suffering.

But water also inflames itching, stirring up alarming paroxysms. The hotter the water, the more intense the seizure. Some sufferers, myself included, allow themselves this means of scratching—not with fingers and nails, but with the hottest water we can stand. Here is fire expressed by its opposite, water, all but burning the skin, inciting a riot of itching, an uproar that just cannot be borne. Comparable to the arc of sexual arousal, the itching increases into the greatest possible concentration, as if at a peak, and then subsides and disappears, sometimes for hours. Doctors say hot water is not good; it opens the blisters and the serum runs. Cold water might be better. But for people constantly restraining their hands from touching the maddening irritation, water brings relief and peace, allowing us to sleep for hours. Though hardly erotic, the course of mounting sensation parallels the later adult rise and fall of desire. To indulge this side of the poison ivy affliction would be to approach a perverse turn in the road. The pain of burning water is so great, however, that usually people do not exploit it for any prolonged erotic taming of distress or inverted satisfaction.

Nonetheless, the coupling of aggression and eros in the itching that hot water arouses, which peaks and then subsides into blissful surcease, enacts and tries to repair a mother's denial of her withdrawal from her child's body. This denial, as Khan says about polymorphous perverse body-experiences, prevents a child from moving "overtly to react with rage and aggression or [to choose] to experience psychically mourning, loss and separateness. Instead the child institutes a dissociation. . . ."[46] Poison ivy forms the battleground for the multiple collisions of opposites. Aggressive attack vies with reaching out so that our plight will be understood by the object. Pain from boiling-hot water contrasts with a pleasing rise and fall of primitive sexual desire. Expressing anger at the loved object conflicts with mourning the object's loss. Longstanding self-holding competes with the disintegration of its condensed textures by yielding to nonintegration, being held in the peace of the bath. The exhibition of a pandemonium of rage, breaking out in skin lesions, fights with acceptance, a letting go to some other source through which mending can advance.

Descending into the bath brings rich archetypal meanings to poison ivy sufferers, none of which I knew as a child when I devised this method of relief. But looking back on my instinctive action of seeking a soothing bath and using fiery water, as well as attacking the itching despite medical prohibition, tells me that my psyche knew something then that my conscious ego-knowing has only since learned. The bath symbolizes a redemption motif. Eleusynian mysteries, Christian baptism, North American Indian sweat lodges—all involve rituals of healing through water. The bathtub represents a human-made vessel, a container that holds the renewing process. In alchemy this contained water was the vessel in which the Philosopher's Stone was made. That the container is invented by humans suggests symbolically that what is learned in the water will be at our disposal, and can be put to conscious use. Plunging into water also means putting the psychological complex back into the unconscious to see what forces work in it. That certainly bore true in my poison ivy events. Rage, pseudosexual arousal, sorrow, all flowed together in the tub. The burning hotness of the water (like Agni, the Indian god of fire) also suggests a sort of conjunction of opposites as conceived by the alchemy of male water and female fire. In its redeemed form, fire acts as a basic image of the Godhead, the tongues of the Pentecostal fire, the light-bringing life, the treasure Prometheus found worth the punishment for stealing to give to humans.[47] Water is also associated with the uterus and the amniotic fluid holding the baby. I remember my surprise when my water broke at the birth of my son. Its temperature was warm, like a bath, the inner bath of the body temperature. We are born from the womb and reborn in rituals of immersion in water. Differentiated from sin or impurities, we emerge from the bath with a new peace, no longer overrun by frenzied destructive mixtures of affects or of personal and collective problems.

Sacrifice

Like any child, poison ivy children come into the world with a capacity for lavish loving. Searles researched this devotion in his early studies of schizophrenia during his nine years at Chestnut Lodge hospital, unearthing a startling fact, he said. Children of schizophrenogenic mothers go crazy because they are unwilling to abandon the parent to the loneliness of a dissociated, archaic state where primitive loving does not differentiate from ruthless aggressiveness. The children sacrifice their sanity in order not to desert their parent. The infamous hateful sparring and verbal annihilations that Searles observed to be characteristic of mother-child couples suffering from schizophrenia, arise not from hate but from love too dangerous to utter. Hateful remarks protected the other from getting too close to the primordial loving which could be destructive.[48]

Poison ivy children partake to a lesser degree in this prodigal sacrifice of self to love of object. Children breathe in what lies around, what has been denied in the family's unconscious atmosphere. For example, my attacks occurred every spring when the ivy bloomed. I would also contract the disease in the fall when the leaves were raked and burned, and sometimes even in the winter from my prowling around the countryside. But springtime brought the annual outbreak of ivy blossoming all over me, almost like a fertility ritual, a sacrifice to the goddess to ensure plenty.

From a conventional point of view, the attacks recurred because of the inevitable contact when the oak, sumac, and ivy flourished. True enough. But in the use the psyche made of the allergy, we can see another quality in its annual recurrence. Yearly, I displayed the anguish I felt as well as the agony transmitted unconsciously in the family atmosphere. It's hard to convey the acuity of this transmission. It is as if the invisible distress underneath the family persona accumulates and boils up, overflowing into visibility through the weeping body of the poison ivy sufferers. Sorrow accompanied my attacks—a wordless, imageless sorrow, a bleak looking into blankness, a seeing that there really could be nothing.

It is not as if this were the only truth and the conscious family behavior was false. Both held truth, but the sorrowful one was denied, given no houseroom, no conscious acknowledgment. That made it immediately infectious, as it floated in the air along with the toxic ivy oil. Just as I was not warned away from the places where ivy grew, the unconscious disappointment and unhappiness were not bounded by anyone dealing with it. Like the ivy that grew in neglected places, the neglected sorrow flourished. Stifled words that needed to be argued through, hindered hopes that no one dared to face, mute inexplicable misery, frustrated talent—all arose, free, ready to be ingested along with the air. A recurring childhood vision of coinciding opposites gives a picture: a perfectly formed circle, large, in shimmering white, beautiful in its wholeness, in the next minute decays, decomposing like Spanish moss, crumbling, fragmenting, shredding into nothingness.

One way I can tell the truth of these words is from the effect on my body when writing this piece. It makes me itch! Spots of poison ivy have turned up on my ankles and arms. A fever has overtaken me, and an aching—as if I have been beaten—makes me take a two-week recess. Internal itching attacked my composure, and a general sickish feeling accompanied my effort to rescue into words the sadness and grieving I experienced when I was responding to my mother's spells of unhappiness and to those of other members of the family as well.

Through some kind of *participation mystique*—unconscious identity between self and other [49]—I not only boiled up and over yearly to bring into plain sight my own conflicts through poison ivy, but also gave expression to what I absorbed as my mother's distress, to join in it, to bring it into visibility, to suffer it on her behalf. It was a kind of sharing between my mother and me, through body care, and it succeeded in showing the distress, thus mending a bit of the schizoid split we suffered. This merging into my mother's unvoiced inchoate pain was a kind of psychic *solutio,* comparable to the actual bath for the sores, and partaking in the alchemical symbolism of that operation. "The *solutio* 'solves' psychological problems by transferring the issue to the realm of feeling . . . it answers the 'unanswerable' questions by dissolving the libido obstruction of which the question was a symptom."[50] The crucial questions remained unanswered because they were never voiced; such questions as: "What are you going through? What is your unhappiness? Why don't you hold me?" All this dissolved into sorrow, resulting in a child's willingness to offer herself in place of the loved one.

The deeper symbolism behind any image of immersion in water, such as the bath, or swimming—to which I was passionately devoted—relates to baptism, "which signifies a cleansing, rejuvenating immersion in an energy and viewpoint transcending the ego, a veritable death and rebirth."[51] The skin of those who suffer poison ivy enacts death and rebirth vividly. Nothing short of miraculous, the inflamed, exploding, weeping, crusted, scarred skin eventually peels off, revealing a fresh, tender container, unmarked like a newborn babe's. The old has been shed and the new has arrived, symbolizing a new beginning and parentage. Like a snake, or its ancient ancestor, the serpent, whose molting configures the perpetual capacity for renewal, the mystery of death and rebirth returns, hovering within the banal and comparatively trivial bout with poison ivy.

The serpent holds ambivalent meaning, as does poison ivy, when each year I shed my skin. The serpent is both poisonous and healing, a preserver and a destroyer, signifying both spiritual and physical rebirth. Related to the masculine with its clearly phallic form, the serpent always accompanies Great Mother deities. Thus the serpent can be seen to suggest the masculine part of the feminine, in Jung's parlance the *animus* potency of the female, here for both my mother and me. In neither of us was this potency tamed. For my mother, outrageous deprivations enforced by her father made her refuse a full four-year scholarship to Wellesley College because it was "charity," and this is but one example. For me, I was still a child, not yet developed in transforming potency into actuality. Insofar as this reconstruction is true, it suggests that lurking in my annual poison ivy festival was an effort to take on my mother's unlived life, shed it, and offer a new beginning. For myself, I was trying to inaugurate a closeness and dependable holding that somehow had been missed, so I could start afresh with a firm foundation, a backing behind me.

The symbolism of the toad proves relevant to the poison ivy sufferer, too. Just as skin exists midway between inner and outer existence, so the toad lives midway between an aquatic and a terrestrial existence. Its skin both separates and links inner and outer worlds, underwater unconscious life and land-based life. It sheds its skin annually. Negatively, the toad can be taken to symbolize dividedness, being split between opposing worlds and committed to neither, but constantly exchanging one for the other; "The skin is then primarily a divider and its casting an act of rejection . . . in which there is a fundamental lack of acceptance of the essential doubleness of life . . . and often with overriding feelings of guilt and fear."[52] Positively, the toad can be seen to symbolize a capacity to live at the frontier of two worlds—the inner and outer, the unconscious and conscious—and remain open to both. Here the toad represents a capacity to be aware of ambivalence and a willingness to participate in many dimensions of existence; it stands for "a position of enlightenment, naturally accompanied by continual regeneration."[53]

The toad's skin is the means by which it receives nourishment, for it both drinks and breathes through it. Thus its skin must always be kept moist. We might hazard a symbolic interpretation, that moist skin means feeling-supplied skin, bathed in a surrounding current of feeling. That was what was denied me in my family atmosphere. My peasant parents were survivors with a toughness that eclipsed their capacity to mourn consciously for their abandoned homeland. But every Sunday I journeyed with them to a nearby city to join other refugees in Slavic language, song, and food, that reincarnated what they all left behind to become American. In addition, this second mother endured the pain of having all her teeth pulled in order to wear dentures. She also endured serious trouble with her bowels; and she never could bear a child. My mother created a hearty atmosphere with her own kind of toughness. She met with pluck and upbeat courage her cancer treatment when I was 12 (much of it alone in another city except for letters I sent her) and when I was 14, her recuperation from a near-fatal car accident that left her in bed for months. No discussion or expression of how hard regaining her health was or of any physical pain ever surfaced in family conversation. My father's feeling-life ran along introverted lines and found its expression in his warm presence to his patients, who often spoke with gratitude of his remarkable healing power, confirmed to me by people speaking about it on the streets of our town, by letters to him, or by sending him books they had written, or giving him hogs they butchered or jams they made. People said they believed when he put his big square hand on them, they must get well. He, too, was in the same near-fatal car accident as my mother. After an initial confinement to hospital, when he would figure out the cubic air-space in my mother's hospital room when visiting her, he quickly returned to work, hiring a nurse to help his wife.

The toad's loose fitting skin represents a proper alternative either to a too uptight "hide-bound" mentality on the one hand or a too loose body-boundary on the other, where unconscious contents or external events can jump into awareness, bringing fear and a sense of invasion, much as the toad startles us with its sudden appearance as it leaps out of a pond. This loose skin retains its containing capacity as long as the toad needs it and can be sloughed off when it is ready. To discard skin, which composes our contact with the outside world around us, can be seen to symbolize an "act of detachment, [from] old worn-out attitudes and loyalty to that which is dead, past and no longer appropriate, so that all life may be experienced freshly, unadulterated by conditioning."[54]

In this sense of shedding the old and generating the new, the skin ritual suggests religious acts. The toad is moved both from within and without to doff its skin. The procedure begins with a "cathartic flow of liquid; takes time and hard work and is carried out in darkness." Reading Dale-Green's description, I think of the endless flow of body fluid that accompanies any bout of poison ivy, as well as the darkened room in which we must lie to spare eyes infected with the serum.

The toad's skin splits "down the middle of the back, exposing the spine, which may be taken symbolically "as a supreme act of differentiation, revealing the central strength." The median down which the skin splits in two could be considered symbolically to represent a third thing, different from what is discarded in two halves. Thus we might hazard that in a poison ivy illness, where skin splits and is discarded, an attempt at differentiation from parental images is taking place, and that the median represents a reuniting of potential opposites. For the toad eats the skin it sloughs off, which might be considered to symbolize the fact that we cannot just evacuate psychic contents in projections and projective identifications onto parents, for that only leaves us vulnerable to their painful repetition. When a toad discards its skin, it then eats the skin, which symbolically can be seen to mean assimilating the contents of a painful complex. Eating is "a powerful expression of interiorization."[55] I don't think I assimilated, that is, "ate" my cast off poison ivy skin until I meditated on the meaning of this repetitious body-compulsion, which is probably the main reason it incessantly repeated itself. The psyche kept using the body's allergy to get my attention, to urge on me the task of metabolizing the emotional experiences poison ivy enacted. And writing about it is an external symbol of the task of internal integration, where "'the slough' continues to live on and, kept inside in an attitude of responsibility and acceptance, it can only increase the power of the whole."[56]

The toad is also associated symbolically to the function of a midwife, who assists in delivering newborn life from an inner to outer state. Heqit, in Egyptian mythology, is depicted as toad-headed, presiding over conception and birth. The pineal eye, seen in the toad's larval stage, and in the adult toad as its third eyelid that enables the toad to see underwater, points symbolically to the "third eye" of spiritual insight. Akin to the *lapis* or the Philosopher's Stone, this eye has been symbolically depicted as a precious jewel, thought to reside in the toad's forehead, representing the newborn spiritual insight the toad helps deliver. Symbolically, the Stone grows in extreme cold, comparable to the "creative chill" of the toad detaching itself from former attitudes and shedding them.[57] The cold might also link to the icy nothingness I felt beneath the surface warmth of my family.

What then did the repetition of poison ivy attacks signify? Why wasn't once enough, especially that attack when I was 10? Is it necessary to drag into image and word the body's eloquent speech in order for meaning to register so that it need not be rehearsed physically every year? Is it impossible to effect meaning unless object and subject grasp it together? Are we so constructed that we cannot really grasp and live spiritual truth unless another also recognizes it and incarnates it? In pondering these questions, a series of dreams about poison ivy, dreamed over the decade after my patient asked his stunning question, hint at the direction of possible answers.

Dreams Again

Four years after the November attack of ivy poisoning, dreams began to play around with the chronic allergy by bringing explicit images of the infection. Shadow figures, not the dream-ego, would turn up with swollen faces or legs. Then I dreamed of a father who, unlike my own, possessed an unpredictable trickster element, offering me medicine that must be taken with milk, which turned out, instead, to be leading me to a woman, with two little daughters, who lived on a boat. This boat existed right in the city's daily traffic, yet in water, thus living both in the known and unknown. In the dream I find my sister is now with me, my shadow side, and we come into the presence of this exotic woman with her lovely girls. The interior of the boat is furnished with richly colored rugs, fine wood, and fabrics. Is this medicine for the bruised and neglected feminine? In both my mother and me? The trickster-father leads us to well-mothered girls, and all of us together make up a total of five, thus recalling the quincunx, the image of my first dream, after the November poison ivy attack that inaugurated this study.

Then a dream came where relief for poison ivy can be found in the medicine cabinet in the hall of my mother's dressing room, suggesting that healing lies in the closets, scents, clothes, and jewelry of a woman attending to her body and femininity. Then I dream my brother gets poison ivy and is to marry a student of mine who is a voluptuous, giving woman—just what he needs. She would confront him and also be very loving. Again, the imagery suggests that the feminine is the restorative balm for the body's infection.

Eight months later (I did not dream about poison ivy all the time!) another strong dream comes. I discover a lethal dose of poison ivy infects my finger and arm, and the dream orders: "You must find its originating point!" I took this task to heart and seven months after that, two dreams depict me with horrendous doses of poison ivy, from ankle to crotch. The ferocious nature of the ivy assault opened me up to the endless weeping expressed in the allergy, and again a threat to my legs. Where could the dream-me stand? A sense of being utterly left with nothing to lean on, stand on, nothing holding me up, flooded into me. Nothing was there, only enough pain to keep me from falling into a void, a gap in being. But soon after came anger, as if to pull me back into life, to personalize the abyss as someone's fault. Dreams of yelling, "I am so mad I could kill you!" at my sister, or a woman friend, ensued. This sequence culminated in another dream, talking with my sister about past lives. She grabs my forearm, infested with poison ivy, and the dream announces: "I had the proof!" Proof of what? I asked on waking. I meditated on the significance of my allergy for my family and the generations of their lives, too. In the dream my infection acts as evidence of *their* vulnerability to being wounded, infected, poisoned, in *their* past as well as present lives.

A year later, the third eye on my forehead turns up again in dream. This time something fiery goes directly into it, penetrating it, uncovering it, finally perhaps allowing it to see. A few weeks later, I saw that the benign neglect of my parents had shifted from something done to me to something I do to myself. In the dream, I have a tiny baby, the size of a nickel (not worth five cents?). I keep going away; it sleeps. When I return, I cannot find it. Where is it! Ah, in the petri dish! The dream announces that the losing and finding of the infant is linked to poison ivy. I felt on waking that my ego finally was pulling the deserted self, unremembered, unheld in anyone's awareness, into my own imagined omnipotence. The unheld baby was now mine to remember and I must awaken to a new task. This bit of beginning life was contained, surrounded by a container specifically designed for new life—the petri dish holding it while it is growing.

Six months later, a dream laid it all out—the etiology, the complexity of opposite emotions, and the way toward cure of the poison ivy miseries. The dream opens in my third-floor childhood bedroom. I am young, no older than 10 because my sister still shares this floor with me. I go into the bathroom, where my sister is bathing and dressing; a small boy is also there brushing his teeth. My mother comes down the hall outside the bathroom and pushes in the bathroom door with a question. I reprimand her for doing so and explain that it is wrong, intrusive to push her way in, and that there is no room in the bathroom. The back of one of my sister's thighs is thick with poison ivy, full of juice, blisters, and sores. When my mother bangs the door in, it bumps against my sister's leg and a big jet of poison ivy juice squirts straight out onto me, which is very dangerous for me. I say this to my mother and try to find some medicine. My sister is not so worried about her own poison ivy.

My sister and I lived on the same floor before I was 10, but in the dream we were adults. That my mother is upstairs suggests a repair of the mother imago and contact with an archetypal mother, because my actual mother rarely came upstairs to my room. This mothering presence makes itself available, coming of its own accord to communicate something to the daughters, albeit intrusively. The dream pictures my ego-capacity to challenge this mother's barging-in style, and not allow her to duck out, to dismiss her own behavior as unimportant. I hold her to it as doing something hurtful and dangerous to me, however inadvertently. Because of her pushing in, I get exposed to the juice that can poison me and interrupt my life for weeks. Poison ivy, then, connects with interrupting the continuity of being, to borrow Winnicott's phrase. The unrelated pushing-in breaks in on my going on being. But the dream-me neither gets in a rage nor withdraws in hurtful isolation, but rather faces the mother's unconscious behavior and makes it conscious to her, a prerequisite to her changing her behavior.

My sister-shadow is attending to her feminine appearance and body, something my actual sister did not take time to do. So attention to the feminine body is increased in this dream; the shadow now cares about her feminine body and beauty. Though infected with poison ivy, she is somewhat blithe about it. Perhaps the dream shows a lighter attitude I could take to the infection; or, perhaps the sister shows the family pattern of denial.

The bathroom is a place of transformation—of dressing, washing, eliminating what needs to be pushed out, and of renewing what is to be conserved. Perhaps the dream-ego should have waited until the sister and the boy were done with their ablutions. He recalls my son when small, symbolizing a lively little masculine presence in touch with mothering females, not veering off unrelated. He brushes his teeth, that is, he takes charge of his own body and his own aggression—cleaning his fangs.

My mother pushes in, but in an unrelated way, which hits my shadow and poisons me. I am hurt through the shadow's body, through my mother unintentionally causing me harm. Her actual harm is in refusing to see that such unrelated behavior brings hurt. She just sticks out her communication without taming it. She is like a woman with a phallus bobbling around, not really owning her masculine potency or aiming it for the purposes she wants to fertilize. Her pattern is to stick out, break in, blurt out, and then dismiss. She needs to put this potency at the disposal of her ego. The dream also shows that the infection that had so waylaid me no longer resides in me, but is located in the sister-shadow. That is progress, even though the place of infection, on the back of the thigh, is hard to see.

The next night after this dream, I dream again of poison ivy, but this time I do not have it or get it, nor does my shadow-sister or anyone else related to me. This time, a young woman, unknown to me (but in the dream the daughter of my aunt), urgently requests an analytic session with me. Seated across from her at a square table, I look out the French doors to a huge square or rectangular swimming pool, almost the length of the building. Her husband and my husband are also seated at the table. I am analyzing her dream, which shows her "picking at Mrs. Blister's blister."

The psyche puts the whole problem out of the personal realm, more or less removed from me, now under my care as an analyst, perhaps reflecting my efforts to analyze the meaning of my body's repetition compulsion. The shape of the table and similar shape of the pool of the unconscious nearby also suggest greater access to the rational meaning of the dream within the dream, as a square symbolizes a defined space for actual grounded living on Earth, by representing limitation—and therefore form.[58] My aunt, my mother's sister, and the wife of the uncle who sang in the opera at my birth, was long and happily married. They were wealthy, lived all over the world because of his singing career, had many friends. My mother envied her and disliked her power-mad antics, but also loved her; she was in her own way much like my mother; she was also a controlling woman.

In the dream, the young woman's husband finds this mother-in-law over-controlling. Both my aunt and mother were complicated women, undifferentiated mixtures of lavish generosity and unconscious power needs. They gave out of their need to unburden themselves of their many gifts, or out of impulse, but without being attuned or matched to the body-rhythms of the recipient. My aunt said to me I should have been her daughter, and her daughter, whom my aunt neglected (benignly) as she traveled around the world with her husband, should have been my mother's child—my mother had cared for her as a little girl and they had remained very fond of one another.

This dream continues the previous poison ivy one, in which the blister on the back of my sister's thigh bursts, aiming poisonous juice straight at the dream-me. Poison ivy produces blisters that we should not pick at, but always do, as they heal. Picking at these blisters is still aggressive behavior turned against ourselves. As an analyst, I would say to this young woman, "Here you are, dreaming your relationship to a controlling but abandoning mother, who also gave lavishly to you, but who did not relate to your body-rhythms. Now you can end up using your aggression against yourself. Though married, your husband is still not yet at ease with the power of his mother-in-law, which is representing that your masculine potency is not yet fully free from your negative mother for your own loving and living. The new point the dream brings is that it is not you who are infected, but this figure called Mrs. Blister, who is not even your own mother, but an archetypal force personified in this infected, negative form. The psyche puts the poison ivy infection outside the family, and puts the mother-daughter problem outside your personal arena, now between a daughter and her own animus, aided by an analyst able to help because she lives in relation to her own animus, symbolized by her own husband." The dream gives an image of the negative source of the illness—the Blister woman. But if the blisters can be picked at, they are on their way to drying up, scabbing, and healing.

The dream figure's concentration on picking at her skin recalled something I had read in Erich Neumann's *The Great Mother*. The Aztecs performed a rite to ensure the fertility of the crops. They sought to transform the chthonic negative power of the unconscious as "mother" from devouring the emerging "son" of consciousness. The rite aimed instead to develop a differentiated conscious ability to relate to nature and the cycles of life.[59] This mother-son transformation of birth into rebirth applies to poison ivy sufferers, too. Feminine giving, from the primordial source of the chthonic mother, must awaken to the conscious ego-discrimination of purpose. It must leave behind the impulse just to flood or barge in on and steal the root impulse of the receiver, as in the previous dream of the mother crowding into the bathroom where her daughters, and with them the accompanying little masculine potency, are cleansing and adorning themselves for conscious living.

In the Aztec ritual, gruesome as it sounds to modern ears, the god Xipe is the masculine equivalent of the chthonic Earth Goddess and also personifies the corn plant that must be sacrificed to give birth to corn, her son. Xipe replaces the Earth Goddess as her "representative on earth" and wears "a short skirt of zapote leaves . . . [and] she is attached to a hole in the middle of the round stone, this hole representing the center and entrance—in the sexual as in other respects."[60] She is sacrificed and her skin flayed; then she is resurrected in her son, which also denotes a kind of sexual congress. The son as priest dons her discarded skin. "The essential elements in this fertility ritual are the beheading of the woman as goddess, the fructifying sacrifice of her blood, the flaying of her body, and the investment of the son-god-priest in her skin."[61]

Skin *is* matter and life-sustaining. To don the skin of the one sacrificed and flayed, whether human or animal (as in Shamanism), is to put on the potency, the mana, of the animal, here the Earth Goddess, and to be put in touch with its instinctive power and knowledge. The new "son" symbolizes victory over the dissolution of the ensnaring unconscious in its personification as a terrible negative mother. As a new young corn god, Xipe represents the life reborn from the destruction and decay of old crops. For poison ivy victims, this ritual sounds a resonating chord. poison ivy patsies are stuck in an ever-recurrent cycle, displaying the suffering of colliding opposites—self-holding versus dependence-on-others, abandonment versus forcing the mother's attention to a young feminine body, helplessness versus assertion, erecting boundaries against the intrusive mother versus needing her containment, rage versus sorrowful weeping over dependencies unmet, making manifest the vision of Nothing versus lavish self-sacrifice to save, or at least join, the other who faces Nothing.

All this misery would be a form, however small, of the ritual of flaying and donning of skin to take on the mana of death issuing in rebirth. To be caught in a mere annual repetition of poison ivy body-speech without arriving at the image-speech of dream or a metaphor that gives voice to meaning[62] leaves us cycling down into the archetypal negative mother. In that downward spiral we fall into stupor (repetition), helplessness (in the grip of the allergy compulsion), enchantment (sacrificing our body for the mother's denied suffering). We get caught in perverse routes to satisfaction (scratching, the pain of the bath) and annihilation (by remaining deaf to the meaning of the body's speech through poison ivy). The beauty of poison ivy, with its luxuriant twining and turning around trees, under brush, over fences, in radiant changing colors, remains, like Dionysus, a parasite dependent on the mother's growth. His potency is sacrificed to the Goddess, just as the affliction of the beautiful ivy captures all its sufferer's energy in rounds of infection, treatment, and endurance.

It is at the bottom of this negative spiral of abandonment and helpless nakedness— we hardly wear much clothing when garbed in blisters!—where poison ivy sufferers feel most exposed to banishment and to the void. It is precisely at this extreme point where the negative shifts and changes into the positive.

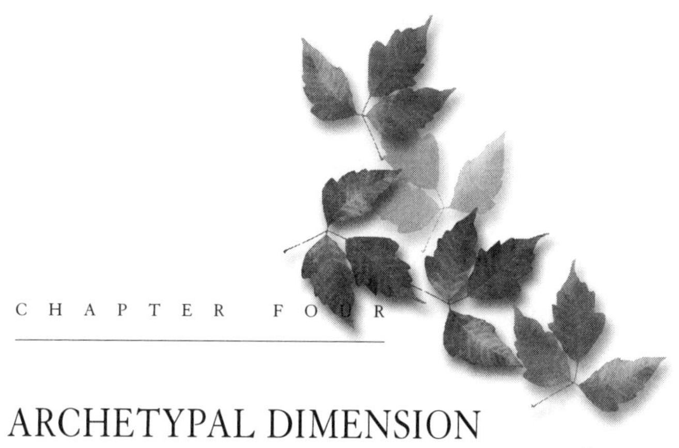

CHAPTER FOUR

THE ARCHETYPAL DIMENSION

If the archetypal situation underlying the illness *can be expressed in the right way the patient is cured . . . shown that his particular ailment is not his ailment only, but a general ailment—even a god's ailment—he is in the company of men and gods, and this knowledge produces a healing effect.*[1]

WITH THESE WORDS, JUNG TRIES TO EXPRESS THE difference it makes to perceive the archetypal dimensions of our illnesses, whether physical or psychic. Three things help: first, to perceive and come to dwell in the liminal space created by the archetypal opposites that collide in poison ivy; from there, healing springs. Second, to enter the sense of shared community that poison ivy ushers us into, as trivial as that itchy problem seems in general, and as excruciating as it is to the various sufferers. A small band of us suffer this affliction. We are the Ivy League: thus we join those who are admitted to select colleges and universities. We are elected to an elite education, elite in the sense of "small in number." We cross the mysterious frontier between body and mind. Third, this sense of community, which supports us in the misery of poison ivy—trading stories, comparing blisters, swapping lotions, bonding as refugees from smooth skins—unites us as transgressors of human boundaries into sacred territory. Are we, as Jung avers, in the company of the gods? Are we sharing God's ailment? The three sources circle round the obscure point of origin of rebirth that springs from the depths of suffering to which this peculiar, stubborn allergy drives us.

The psyche makes use of this somatic nadir to scout its own vision of meanings assembling on the horizon. The gathering meanings show several themes: from obscure slime, the sublime inaugurates its own shape; our dependency upon each other is lifelong and must not be denied; if accepted, it blooms into interdependency. The divine, or whatever we call the reality that transcends both psyche and soma, which communicates its *numen* through the archetypal dimension of the psyche, wants to step over into concrete human life. The divine looks to incarnate.

Opposites and Liminal Space

"Archetypal" is a word pointing to the dimension of human experience that falls outside ego-consciousness. It originates elsewhere and thus cannot be fully known, or at least known in advance, by the ego.[2] That fact makes the ego uneasy. We feel the burden of something being pushed for, but we do not know for certain what it is, or who is doing the shoving. Jung suggests we give a name to this factor, whose derivatives turn up in our conscious experience, in order better to relate to it. Better to call it a god than just what I ate for dinner last night, or a phobia.[3] Consciousness protects us from mania and evokes proper respect. We humbly recognize that we are involved with some great presence, or rather, that it involves itself with us, lest we lapse back into the idea that we know all about it and really remain in charge.

Another way Jung describes this presence transcending the whole psyche, turns round the psyche's use of archetypal symbols to communicate the reality to us. Archetypes are "the tools of God."[4] A rough map of the levels of psychic reality that transgress ego-consciousness is helpful here. At the deepest core, far down inside us and far outside us dwells the radically free, unfathomable, ever-present transcendent reality that we call God, or that we deny when we say there is no God. At the next level, working up toward ego-consciousness, archetypes exist as contents of the collective unconscious, that level of the psyche shared by all humanity, though packaged differently in different cultures and historical periods. Above this collective layer of the objective psyche, so to speak, the individual soul exists, which Jung understands as the function of relationship between our conscious ego and the inaccessible depths of the unconscious.[5] Our souls reflect up to consciousness images of the archetypes and down to the collective unconscious the effects of consciousness (including our shared cultural consciousness). The result of these opposite poles meeting is our construction of symbols.

In the space of the radical commerce of transferences between individual and collective traditions, our originality is born. The soul is like a two-way mirror, reflecting both the unconscious and what addresses us through the unconscious to the ego, and what addresses the unconscious through our ego, including collective ego-awareness, the regnant images and thought forms of our time. Our souls register and express the reality that transcends both consciousness and unconsciousness, a reality that addresses us and acts on us through the instrumentation of the archetypes and through the agency of ego-life, both personal and shared in our culture.

Our souls spontaneously create symbols to register our experience of this transcendent action in "an image that describes in the best possible way the dimly discerned nature of the spirit. A symbol does not define or explain; it points beyond itself to a meaning that is darkly divined yet still beyond our grasp, and cannot be adequately expressed in the familiar words of our language."[6] Such symbols are "inexhaustible" because they are not "objects of the mind, but categories of the imagination which we can formulate in ten thousand different ways . . . they are *before* the mind, the basis of everything mental."[7]

Our project here, ridiculous as it may sound, is to inquire into the symbolic meaning of the chronic poison ivy allergy. What use does the psyche make of this bodily affliction to communicate something that transcends ego awareness? And, if it is a true symbol, what is it that cannot be better expressed than in this way, through body-language? Body-speech, as I have said, is remarkably communicative if we have ears to hear. We must not treat it as a "lower" form of animal life which we will "rescue" into human words. It is precisely this animal life, this organ-dialect, that forms the stuff of the symbol in poison ivy. Skin gathers up multiple meanings, as we have seen, frontiers—between physis and psyche, between child and parent, between inner life and outer world, in all the many emotional opposites explored above. What more tidy sum is there than the body's terse eloquence! It has taken pages to elaborate the implicit meanings of this skin distress. The body-ego's somatic consciousness has borne the responsibility to communicate the idea that is so eager to be incarnated, and whose "corset" brought me to an ability to house nonbeing within my own physical limits.

The effect of this allergy that the psyche exaggerated in order to express conflicts of my own, and conflicts within my family, and through these means all human conflicts, is to create a space between a body riddled with blisters and an awareness of their meaning. For me, a sort of no-man's land came to exist in that shadowed room, in the lotion rituals, in the middle of the night when I would soothe the discomfort with the dulling powers of oatmeal in the bathwater. I was definitely flesh and not yet spirit, but living both in time out of time, plucked out of my childhood round of play, homework, and family life. Confined to bed, no longer ranging through the countryside, no longer with the animals, not even the human ones of my family, I lay there drifting, nowhere, a nothing.

Slowly that space took on liminal tones, like the *kairos* time of a yearly ritual. This space granted me time out from the unconscious assumption of responsibility for carrying unhappiness that was lying around me in the atmosphere. Poison ivy framed some weeks to put that burden down, and to show it forth instead, not to metabolize it into my system. Poison ivy was an effort to flush that unhappiness out of my system, to be rid of it. Yet it was also a reiterated urge to individuate: "the purpose of the psychosomatic symptom must reflect the overarching purpose of the Self, which is to direct the process of individuation . . . the psychosomatic symptom cries to be relieved, it cannot be fixed. Its irrational nature can only be resonated with empathically."[8]

The world around me still existed, but I was not in it. I was marginalized, taken to the frontier outlined by my skin. For some weeks, my ordinary world desconstructed and chaos supervened. Sleep was interrupted so I could itch and scratch and bathe and put on bandages; daytime was darkened, with curtains half-drawn; skin erupted; mother, so distant, appeared with periodic regularity; unconscious suffering displayed itself right out in the open: the body wept and raged and wept. I exhibited the ugliness, usually covered up, of denied frustrations and sadnesses infiltrating the atmosphere. I incarnated them deep down in my body.

A liminal space grew up during these poison ivy fests that were both reiterations of the old plight and reachings for a new beginning. By the time healing arrived, I was, like a snake, shedding the old skin to reenter the world with a new hide. Slowly, over the years, I built up capacities—to stand and relieve pain, and process it, to house nonbeing, to rest from some intercessory role I had taken on unwittingly, to grab my own sanity and quit those who did not join me. Poison ivy became a space of transition, where opposites collided as well as differentiated. My ego bogged down in repetition of the allergy, and then, with this present effort to express the meaning of poison ivy, slowly gained some flexibility. Psyche using body gives way to space between them where their conversation occurs.

Our ego is the one who makes the transition, from repetition compulsion to a ritualized acknowledgment of psychic reality. When our ego-space enlarges to accommodate the play of our reflection upon the dense interlockings of flesh and spirit, it moves to more fluid articulations of each dimension, and makes easier their conjoining. What we suffer psychically does not always need to be suffered physically, as the remarkable cessation of the outbreak of the allergy since I began my musings on it indicates. We are astonished by how slow we are, how finite finitude is. We construct a space so these colliding, coinciding opposites can be seen together in their complexity. What grows out of it and builds within its shelter, does so very slowly. Nonetheless it grows, steadily, too—the new body of the snake in its new skin.

Jung writes about the "breath body" that "rises out of our coarse body and floats in the air . . . that middle thing which the primitives call 'the subtle body' . . . which is spirit as well as body. It is the union of the two by this thing between."[9] Similarly, in the myth of Marsyas, the story tells of preserving his skin after it is stripped off his body. His skin is pierced like Christ's, cut off in order to empty it of its blood. The protective envelope is torn from him. But then his skin is preserved to make an impenetrable shield, mighty in its safeguarding capacity, like the goat skin Athene used as immunity in conquering the giant Pallas, or the skin of Achilles rendered invulnerable by his goddess-mother, like the golden fleece originally offered by Zeus to keep two children safe from their stepmother's murderous intentions.[10]

The fragile ego, embedded in matter, suffering its enmeshment in the poisoned body, somehow locates itself in the space intermediate between body and mind that is needed for any healing transformation. The ego finds refuge in this space created by the ceaseless play of the psyche—elaborating, embellishing, unfolding, improvising, augmenting, conserving our experience, while creating and finding its meaning. Our ego is needed to incarnate the idea that seeks expression. To mediate the something beyond the ego into concrete living, it must go through the ego, be housed by the person. Otherwise, the ego is just felled, or left out of it. Then we endure psychosomatic symptoms in which the body is burdened and the ego is bypassed. Symbols rise and fall; numinous archetypal events happen and cease. Nothing changes. Like a shuttlecock, one is batted back and forth, now out of contact with the ivy, sumac, oak divisions, now in contact with them and contracting, in both senses of the word, a period of indenture.

Still another possibility that omits the ego comes from the archetypal mana substituting for ego-consciousness. Our ego just steps aside, blanks out, or never emerges in the first place. Archetypal energy occupies the place where we should be conscious. Then we fall victim to the outsized power of the archetype, a larger-than-life manifestation of unconscious and unhumanized energy. Instead of being just the mother of this or that child, or a motherly influence upon this group of people, we whoosh into being "The Mother" to everybody. And we brook no interference with expending this virtue in all directions, wanted or not. We rush aloft like a helium balloon, inflated beyond our proper size, or just as suddenly deflated, crashing down, bruised, broken.

The hanging of Marsyas on the tree sounds a note like the ordeal of those of us who suffer poison ivy infestation. One is helpless, lying abed, hoping not to stir the wind, lest itching fly in. The Christ figure on the cross symbolizes helplessness of the ego, and its necessary submission and willing surrender to what transcends it. This broken body completely opposes what in the Roman age reigned as god, that is, power. The cross purposes of that age—and ours—come to a dead stop in that hanging figure. All the petty and gigantic meanness that one human can do to another come to a full halt in the innocent Christ who suffers as if guilty. As the philosopher-theologian Jean-Luc Marion put it so pithily, in Christ is announced: evil stops here.

Christ arrests the inexhaustible logic of evil, where one assault breeds the next, where we first protest our innocence of fault and our undeserving injury, and then feel justified in our anger at being attacked and attacking in return. We feel vindicated in our impulse to revenge, to retaliate against someone, so that finally we reason we have a right to injure, insult, betray, malign, and finally kill the other.[11] Christ takes all meanness and its attendant suffering into himself and ends it there. He, though innocent, suffers all guilt. Evil stops dead in him. All suffering defeats our ego and can rescue us into another dimension beyond itself, but only if we yield, give into, give over to the transcendent unknown meanings, beyond ourselves.

The myths of the hanging gods (Christ, Dionysus, Attis, Mithra, Marsyas, Odin) those hanging on the tree of life done up as cross, symbolize the inevitable coincidence and collision of life's opposites, and touch any suffering we endure, however tiny or great. These figures, and Christ above all, traverse the arc that opposites describe, that just turn up at the same time, as a striking coincidence, in, for example, the death of a parent when a child marries, or the birth of a tough lasting relationship that emerges out of the death of a child, or the death of a relationship that cannot sustain the birth of a child. This coincidence of opposites often enough turns into their collision, into a conflict of opposites. Love vies with hate for the same good person in our lives; simultaneously we feel dependent and assertive. We want to diet and give way to greedy gobbling. We work out a strategy for peace, but it also excites warlike retaliation.

Environmental protective measures we endorse also threaten people's needed jobs. We seek to be kind and out jump hostile remarks; we are going to give up drink, but not just yet. We are felled by the intricate, dense complexity of opposites; we cannot escape their simultaneous appearance and rounds of conflict. The more we see into their dynamics, the more impressive their interweaving. With enough strife, and the mysterious construction of liminal space intermediate between the opposites, we begin to see how the opposites might conjoin and converse. Instead of canceling out each other, they begin to appear as a frame for this transitional space in which are housed a growing sense of self and symbols for what transcends it.

From this rather abstract and exalted note, back to the concrete and small—the poison ivy sufferer. Not until I asked the question, thanks to my patient's prompting, of what meaning the recurrent attacks of poison ivy could bring me, did the repetition open to grow into this space and the attacks cease. That miracle of cessation still impresses me, though I do not challenge it by reckless exposure to the plant. Neither do I cringe. I just take the usual precautions, nothing excessive, nothing different really from what I have always done. The body has grown a protective immunity. After fifty years! Thus the slowness and limits of the ego impress themselves upon us—how small it is, how finite its finite resources. And how necessary. We need our finite consciousness to incarnate and submit to what transcends us. For mediating of the transcendent to occur, we must have an ego to receive the symbol's mediation, and there must be something there which can get mediated and do the healing.

Community

One of the outstanding conflicts of opposites, in whose tensions Otto Rank located his entire depth psychology, his contrast of life-fear with death-fear and of the neurotic with the artist, boils up between our instinct for uniqueness and our need to belong to the herd. We want to be like each other, to imitate what we admire and even what we fear. Yet the urge to realize all of ourselves, to be who we are meant to become, clashes with our need to belong. Yet we can only really relate to others if we can bring our uniqueness into direct connection with theirs.[12] In Jung's thought, individuation contrasts sharply with individualism—the realization of self at the expense of others. Becoming all of oneself (individuation), with all the parts, ugly, undeveloped, as well as superior and skilled, can only occur in relation to each other and to the collective, which is to say to the group, to society, to the human family.

The nothing-place where my annual poison ivy retreats dropped me, became liminal space. It plucked me out of singular confinement in my own body. At the same time, it plunged me into it; it ushered me beyond the small circle of immediate family into a bigger alliance that only recently I have come to call the Ivy League. That select group, elite in size, elected through suffering rather than accomplishment, through lack of protective shield rather than for excellence of defense, brought unexpected comfort. All the members recognize each other. I felt an increased bond with my South Carolina patient who spoke of her battle with the disease when rushed to the hospital. Empathy filled me for a stranger, when I heard about a friend of his who suffered greatly for two weeks in a hospital after his induction into the ivy clan. I mistook the bad scars on another friend's leg one summer when he arrived on a hot day in shorts as the remnants of a sumac rampage, only to learn they lingered from childhood burns. That told me how deep ivy lesions can go, that I could mistake them for something much more serious. That we are not all alone in the adversity of the chronic ivy allergy brings comfort. Others bear the same kinds of marks on their bodies. Shared calamities relieve shame. Instead of being singled out and then isolated, a whole band of fellow-sufferers share the same fate. That community transcends our immediate environment. I may be the only member of my family confined to this yearly time-out, but others beyond my family partake of the same violent recess.

Community, we thus learn, transcends time and place. We can feel common bonds with those we do not know and do not see who share the same searing experience. Oddly enough, then, that liminal space, where we make the transition into the intermediate realm between body and mind, self and other, symbol and reality, turns out to be populated by many such voyagers. What begins as imaginary, takes on spiritual substance. Good and true neighbors exist.

Joining this invisible community weakens the dogged undercurrent of suspicion that somehow we have caused this misfortune that so inconveniences everyone. Judeo-Christian tradition explores this murky underworld of blame and guilt in the examination of the scandal of sin. Wasn't this man born blind because he sinned? Or because his parents sinned? So the disciples ask Jesus (John 9:1-3). Or, on some unconscious level, does ivy repeatedly poison me because I am bad? Is my itching really unexploded anger? Is it my fault that my mother is unhappy because when I was born multiple sadnesses befell her? Does festering skin prove I am the crazy one? Beneath our family's surface happiness, which clearly exists, does another realm of woeful lament and nullity abide even though no one else seems to notice it? Do blisters infiltrate my skin because I know about this other realm? And should I not be noticing it but, instead, be denying it, pretending it isn't there, as others seem to do?

To discover from the American Academy of Dermatology that poison ivy, oak, and sumac as a conglomerate danger affect nine to fifteen million Americans every year, and potentially many more if it were to expand to the world population, brings heartening news. I am no longer stuck in glorious isolation! The scandal of sin cannot be reduced to the scandal of fault. The disease exists objectively. Others share it. Community relieves us of fantasies of omnipotence, even if only negative ones. That frees up aggression for personal use.

When we see our fear of power to cause harm amounts to just that—fear—we need no longer withdraw from spontaneous aggression in order to save the children of the world, or our unfulfilled mothers. To be trapped in omnipotence, whether in inflation or deflation, sets us on a tense itinerary devoid of the resources of aggressive energy and imagination. To be released from the deep worry that somehow we are at fault for the other's misery is like being let out of school or jail. The day beckons. We hand the world back to Atlas. We just must carry our own small part, not the entire globe.

Those of us sustaining the ordeal of our small portion of the poison ivy allergy, can feel part of a bigger society, members of the League. To be relieved of isolation in order to participate in reality with others brings with it ethical obligations. I felt that prodding in the ten years of meditating on poison ivy. What could I learn, I asked myself, that might prove useful to members of our ivy guild? This tie forms another layer of community. In addition to the immediate neighbor with whom we compare scars, remedies, procedures for recovery in a swapping of information and telling of stories, there are others whom we never see who are in the clan. This unseen, even secret group suggests another meaning of "elite." This club of people knows about the connection through psychic reality, soul reality. By looking into ourselves, instead of just at ourselves, we look to the originating point outside ourselves as well as outside our ego-consciousness. By everyone looking *there*, we form a bond *here*. Our connection forms not through knowing each other, but through each of us looking to the same originating point. Enacting obligation to that point forms the ethical life of the group, and circulates energy among us.

That point is the *arché*, the absolute beginning that originates the movement that in turn creates a line, which, as the line moves, creates a plane, and when the plane moves forms a solid, and when the solid moves creates space and time.[13] To see the archetypal dimension of something even as small as poison ivy, allows us to see through all things, big and little, to the point of origin. The point is a central image of the reality transcending the psyche from which all things flow. Jung refers to it in the symbols of fire and light, the *scintilla*; the spark shining in the primordial stuff of life.

To see the *arché*, to see the *scintilla*, to apprehend this archetypal dimension of the psyche and of problems such as poison ivy, through which unfathomable reality draws near enough to be fathomed, allows us to see our psychic life objectively. Aggression freed from fantasy and the fear of omnipotence gives life to this "ruthless self-knowledge."[14] The actual living process goes on in me, in my subjectivity, but remains itself; it addresses me and solicits my participation. We see what is there, like a river flowing through us. We do not put it there. The river takes its source from outside us, but nonetheless flows through all the intimate personal places of our living. We know we did not make the river. Disidentifying with it, we are free from demoralization, from the conviction, for example, that the poison ivy repetition is our "fault." When our energy is not diverted into guilt, it supplies the stamina for seeing into and contemplating the reality beyond us that lives in us even in our illness.

Dreams Again

There are strong examples of seeing through the personal to the transpersonal, of ruthlessly differentiating ego from archetype, where our subjective ego functions to perceive and transmit, and the archetypal depth of psyche functions to display objectively what is there flowing through us. The following dreams show what I mean. The first two arrived on consecutive nights. (I had already dreamt the dream of the lost mother and of directly suffering poison ivy. See pages 77–78). I dreamed that I am for the first time in black with a headdress of a little chair or deer horns, ready to take intitiatory orders. The next night, I dreamt a vicious shadow figure invades my working space and attacks me with condemning remarks. But she won't sit still long enough to answer my confronting her and fighting. She walks around getting cakes or cookies and will not be pinned down. Another woman with her is more passive and the dream-me confronts her. But then they disappear! It is not clear if this is evasion or if I have vanquished them. But my face and neck are red and swelling with a bad case of poison ivy, hurting.

On awakening, I thought the attack, the too-sweet diet and the poison ivy pain, especially in the throat chakra where head joins chest, connected some aggressive depreciating of me, or a denial of it with a too-sweet attitude and the outbreak of painful ivy-poisoning. The throat, which is the organ of speech, symbolizes speaking out, communicating the inner self to outer world, and it hurts. This descent into pain and defense follows the initiation of wearing the headdress (the chair associates sometimes to cow-horns of Hathor; and it could also be reindeer horns). Two years later, I dreamt again of the reindeer and recalled its earlier appearance; this later dream showed a deer, with horns, feminine, coming to me and I know I am going to sit leaning on it as I proofread eighty pages of a manuscript. Also a white polar bear is around and two more animals, four in all.

Hathor, in Egyptian symbolism, was thought to be the mother of the sun-god until Isis replaced her. Sometimes she was identified with the sun, "wearing on her head the sun-disc flanked by a cow's horns" because she was thought to raise the sun up to its place in the heavens by means of her horns. She was "regarded as the solar eye." She was a sky goddess and depicted in bovine form, as the sky was pictured then to be a cow. She was worshiped "as female soul with two faces"—heavenly and also as a goddess of the dying person who followed the setting of the sun.[15] The feminine reindeer bearing horns, possible to both sexes, represents in Lapland the feminine spirit that can pick her way through wilderness and cold to find nourishment. She is a free, independent spirit, sturdy yet delicate, thought to link heaven and earth, a true psychopomp. My dreams thus spoke of hostile aggression connected to poisoning by the ivy and a defense of sweetness that needed to be confronted. The attack of condemnation, that is, making me feel small, a kind of moral sadism, leaves me with poison ivy. But the dream shows that the dream-me is also initiated into this insight and into the rising and dying behind it; that is, I am capable of becoming conscious of the poisonous self-judgment that contaminates sweetness by misusing it. See through this, carry to it the sun of consciousness the dream seems to be saying, to perceive the transpersonal aspect of the death and displacement this sequence imposes. The later reindeer dream suggests a more sure connection to the feminine spirit, sturdy yet delicate, a psychopomp, on which I can depend, that was only begun in the earlier inititating dream. The manuscript was one I was finishing about a brave woman facing dying and what presented itself to her from the other side.[16] She dreamt of an archetypal feminine spirit heralding her death and where she would arrive—a green and pleasant land.

Two years later, I dreamt two dreams that confirmed this tie to the archetypal feminine. They arrived two days apart and four years after the November attack of poison ivy that initiated this study.

In the first dream I am lying down in a circular skiff which rushes off the terrace and swiftly into the pond, hitting the water with a big bang. The shock of the blow rings from the back of my head down to my coccyx, jolting me awake.

In the second dream, which came two days later, I see a young woman, who falls backward down a well, bangs from head to tail against the wall, and gets stuck, hanging by one foot upside down in the well. The dream-me races up to help her and then to tell a nearby man and a woman to get help. Then I run down again to see how she is doing. I see she has gotten free, but I know I had seen, as if I myself had been hanging upside down by my foot, that beneath her a white flame or *fleur de lis* that lives there in the bottom of the well is just coming into bloom.

In my association, I knew the girl was college age, a time for me of facing the abyss, the nothing-place, what poison ivy also threw me into. The hanging upside down recalled the "hanging man" of tarot cards, whose inversion symbolizes a radically changed perspective, inscribing on consciousness the relativity of things, depending on which way you look at it. The old view, if insisted upon, goes bankrupt as the figure's emptying wallets indicate on the tarot card. But the figure's tranquil expression on the card indicates that he has accepted the situation; he represents the gaining of a new view on life, of a change of vision. The picture depicts a moment of transition, from one view to its opposite. Much like one of the hanging gods, the tarot picture shows the ego held in suspense; its view is turned upside down. Death of the old way of looking at things is proclaimed, and a new one granted, if accepted. The tree, though still alive, with its cut-off limbs and in the shape of a Tau cross, indicates the tree of sacrifice. The figure is not dead but suspended, and suggests, with the nimbus around the figure's head, a great awakening. After the mystery of death of an old perspective, a mystery of ressurrection comes, and this is the originating point for a new way of seeing things.[17]

The dream does not show clearly which foot the woman hangs from, probably her left, but looked at from the viewer's perspective, it could be the right. So even the figure herself conveys the coincidence of opposite perspectives, depending on whether we look out from her vantage point or from ours. If she hangs from her right foot, that suggests a hiatus, an abeyance of consciousness with its accustomed ways of seeing and doing; if from the left, then the unconscious standpoint and its customary link to the feminine is where she hangs from. I tend to favor the left foot because it is a woman hanging, unlike the tarot card figure, and the personal associations of college and poison ivy knit this figure with my own struggles. In addition, both the hanging dream-girl and the dream-ego behold a symbol of feminine depth and power.

The white flame of the *fleur de lis*, as a stylized lotus or lily, symbolizes both the Queen of Heaven and the triple majesty of God in the Trinity because of its phallic shape. Yet this flower blossoms deep down in a well, a sort of depth trinity, not the exalted heavenly God, but perhaps the earthy female trinity of Diana, Hecate, and Selene. After all, I spent most of my youth not unlike Diana, roaming the fields, woods, and brooks of the countryside; and I knew firsthand the abyss of Hecate's underworld; and the feminine light of Selene, goddess of the moon, bore great similarity to the distant paleness of the feminine shining toward me from both of my mothers. They were more like warriors than anything else, both of them strong, brave, intrusive, but on the feminine side more fragile, suffering unfulfillment. Both had lost their minds' hold on reality before death. The flower depicts a feminine circle combined with a masculine trinity, associated with the kings of France and military power.[18] Flame symbolically associates with the Holy Ghost of the Pentecost, to inspire fiery speech that communicates across all usual barriers.[19]

The flower is shown both to the dreamer and to the hanging young woman, who merge at the end of the dream. What did I make of it? The dream pressed itself into me. It said to me that under the mother complex something else of numinous presence and power dwelt. In both dreams the psyche bangs on my body to get my attention and wake me up to the momentous reality that under the mother complex, down at the bottom of its abyss which is now a contained well, lives the white flower-flame of regeneration and transformation. Turned upside down, the part of me that faces the abyss sees what shines through it. Our complexes matter; they form the *materia* through which we work through our salvation or fate, or, through which fate works us. If we accept our complexes, and struggle with them, they give us the means through which we work out our salvation, the salvation offered us. But our complexes are not final. Rather, our personal problems form the means that bring us to see what communicates to us through them.

Our seeing, naming, and now living in relation to what speaks through the complexes redeems them. They function to deliver us where we belong. Jung describes this ruthless urge to individuate when quoting the alchemist Gerhard Dorn: "This objective knowledge of the self . . . [means] . . . no one can know himself unless he knows *what*, and not *who*, he is, on what he depends, or whose he is . . . and for what end he is made."[20] Jung finds Dorn's distinction between "quis" and "quid" to point to the distinction and relation between ego and Self: "whereas 'quis' has an umistakeably personal aspect and refers to the ego, 'quid' is neuter, predicating . . . an object which is not endowed even with personality. Not the subjective ego-consciousness of the psyche is meant, but the psyche itself as the unknown . . . 'what' refers to the neutral self, the objective fact of totality, since the ego is...causally 'dependent on' or 'belongs to' it, and . . . is directed to it as to a goal. This recalls the impressive opening sentence of Ignatius Loyola's 'Foundation': 'Man was created to praise, do reverence to, and serve God our Lord, and thereby to save his soul.'"[21]

This dream showed me I belonged to the archetypal feminine, to the mother-flower-flame which I discovered through my experiences with my own mothers. The flowering flame is given to all of us, an image of the unseen energy in existence, the fire of the Holy Ghost, the manifestation of spirit in body. Without denying the particulars of my mothers and me, we were set in a bigger base. That is the difference the archetypal dimension makes. It grants our personal life more room. It plants us in deeper soil with ample room for our roots to grow.

Slime and the Stone

Different strands weave together from this study. Both psyche and body must be included for us to grasp the possible meanings of a chronic, serious poison ivy allergy. Analysis gives us the power to hear this body-speech. The archetypal dimension of psyche and the reality its symbols point to usher us, not only into the company of each other whose community brings solace to our ill state, but further, into the company of the gods where we can see that even our illnesses make a bridge to the transcendent. Conducted *there*, glimpsing the divine, heals us *here*. Relieved either of the disease or of its isolating power, we see through its ministrations that we are already living in this other time which is out of time, in the liminal space with another presence that transcends us. Surely that is what Saint Paul meant when he sounded those glorious words that nothing could separate us from God in Christ, neither death nor life, neither principalities nor powers (Romans 8:38).

But how do we know this? Let us return to the small, the poison ivy league. The body thinks up this allergic way of working on affliction, an allergy which can be avoided because it is not psychosomatic, but somehow is not evaded because the psyche needs make use of it. The body devises its own organ-speech to express wretchedness and to heal it, but on a yearly basis. The very repetition calls attention to itself, bidding us to look for the unknown "X," that extra something that overdetermines the natural, forcing it into the reiterated.

Unearthing the archetypal situation underlying the illness opens the way to community with fellow sufferers and with the transcendent. Poison ivy symbolizes the basic skin-container breaking down, breaking out, breaking through to a larger, more objective, container, encompassing the lacunae suffered by a particular family or a specific mother-child couple. The skin as container in poison ivy is too small and we ask too much of it—to develop prematurely a self-holding in place of resting on another's lap or in another's arms. This premature solution breaks down and communicates a child's gesture to be held and the child's gesture toward holding for the parent what lies denied in the unconscious. The ailment is one of heart energy and the solution is found in *solutio*, dissolving back into feeling, whatever it may be—rage, empathy, arousal, woe, or despair.

Many theorists want to call body-language presymbolic and find curative elements through translation into words or imagery. This is no doubt true. But the eloquence of body-speech takes us further. It communicates in the round, so to speak. Affect, sensation, body-thinking, and the perception of others combine to speak through body-presence, all of a whole round piece, brought alive by fluctuations of mood, gestures of limb, glances of eye, postures of spine. We must not rank body-speech as lower on some artificial scale of progress. It is not "pre-" anything. It is itself. Part of the meaning of poison ivy pulls us down into the body, which says all that needs to be said.

Poison ivy in its gooey, gushy aspects returns its sufferers to the state of primordial slime from which we and all our functions emerge. Jung says, "no individuation can take place . . . without the animal, a very dark animal coming up from primordial slime, enters [sic] the region of the spirit; that one black spot, which is the earth, is absolutely indispensable on the bright shield of spirituality."[22] The completeness of body-speech mirrors in its archaic symbolism the inchoate experience we reach of the trans-symbolic, of reality that surpasses our ability to grasp it in image or word. In both states we suffer confusion in the sense of nonintegration, in the sense of the ego not reigning supreme, but rather being left in a disorganization of plenty. The overflow, the abundance of as yet uncoordinated impulses, of snippets of affect and random thoughts, of fugitive images and embryonic insights, does not fit tidily into an imaginative scheme or into words. Poets live right there on the edge of that profusion, working to find words pregnant or hollow enough to house this plenty in communicable ways without reducing it to finite size.

Right there we pause. We are delivered right there, on the borders of the containing skin of this plenty. Unlike animals, whose instinct perfectly aligns them with the impulse of energy into behavior, we humans hesitate, pause, experience hiatus.[23] Our nature inhabits this gap, and we suffer it as a void if we fall into it. But if supported by another, we enter the gap as the space between, intermediate between psyche and physis, imagination and external world, self and other, between self to be found and one to be created, the liminal transitional space where symbols are born. The gap opens onto the plenty that reality bestows. Our specific task as humans centers on reflecting on what is there, creating it, finding it, sharing it, working our imaginations upon it. We elaborate it and our selves unfold through it in countless varied ways as expressions of our joy and gratitude for the life given us.

But who is the donor? From whom do the gifts stream forth? With whom are we engaging in this radical commerce? Who is the author of the community that grows up when we all look toward the same horizon to see what shows itself there? Who dwells behind the manifold varieties of representation of that presence? If we accept the archetypal dimensions as categories of looking and listening when working with our own complexes, as analysts do with their analysands, then these questions inevitably impose themselves. When Jung says that even our illnesses may partake of the numinous, or our illnesses may even participate in "a god's ailment," then the accent falls on how we relate to the numinous. What is our approach to it? How are we responding or failing to respond to its approach?

Here we see that at both ends of our lives, from our earliest undifferentiated efforts to respond to and give form to our experience of life, from our "slimehood" so to speak, as well as from our most developed articulation and presentiment of what life means, that this other, this transcendent that we sense, exceeds our human grasp. It dwells in radical freedom, always confounding our formulations of its nature, bouncing out of definition, breaking up words by its own hard-as-rock reality.

A symbol for this "other" that garners both a commonplace ubiquity, to be stumbled over by anyone at any place, and a rare, prized, unique presence, is the stone. Stones are both base pebbles and rare gems. Children hide small stones as Jung did a black one in his pencil box, or as a woman analysand of mine did in burying a bright blue stone in a vulva-shaped opening in a cement pavement.[24] These children treat their stones like hidden treasures to be safeguarded at all costs—sacred secrets. The stones, we surmise, represent a core of true self, hidden away, safe from trespassing impingements that threaten their integrity. By tradition, the stone marks the sacred. Examples abound, like the gigantic monuments to cosmic forces as at Stonehenge, in Jacob's altar of stones for Yahweh's angel, in Islam's Ka'bah, the black stone in its holiest shrine at Mecca. The stone of stones that the alchemists constructed and called the Philosopher's Stone, the *lapis*, represents God within the human personality. The living stone of the New Testament is the one on which the church is grounded and to which Peter invites us when he says : "So come to him, to the living stone which was rejected by men but chosen by God and of great worth to him. You also, as living stones, must be built up into a spiritual temple . . ." (1 Peter 2:4).[25]

Poison ivy, as I have known it, is surely an illness touching psyche as well as body. It opened up its own path to this transcendent realm. Like any very hard experience that befalls us, if we wrestle with it time and again we may win through to the obdurate and resolute kernel of truth at its core. If so, that suffering experience confers on us a blessing. The blessing, like an imperishable stone that we take with us the rest of our lives, amounts to the adamantine truth that we have discovered for ourselves. We participate in the originating point. We enter the domain of that author whose work eludes our grasp but always gives forth and accompanies us. The symbol of the stone, so immovable, so imperishable, so common, so precious, symbolizes the presence of this other. We cannot define this other but only describe our experience of its presence.

My first dream after the patient's stunning question to me about the meaning of this allergy gave an objective reading of the situation, which I am still trying to humanize and incarnate into life fully lived, though the dream is over ten years old. The five-sided quincunx, symbolizing realization in life, grounding in living, not just abstract form, is pushed down into a circular shaft. Is it my esophagus? Am I to swallow, to digest, to make part of my flesh this abstract symbol of wholeness? This archetypal perspective does not bring much comfort or enlightenment to immediate suffering. It certainly seemed a far cry from the mundane itchings of poison ivy. But the archetypal symbols of quincunx and circle into which it is pressed do bring a totally different perspective, a picture of what is going on from the psyche's point of view. That new perspective invites the exercise of the human gift for hiatus, for pause, for reflection and inquiry into meaning. This effort helps assemble whatever meaning that will show itself coming over the horizon.

The dream says that the meaning is like pushing a five-pointed shape down a circular shaft. The dream gives a picture of that meaning. But who took this picture? That question takes us through the layers of psyche—my personal experience with my analysand's question, my history with poison ivy, the psyche's abstract symbol of what is objectively happening—to a point of origin beyond both personal and archetypal dimensions. In the large arc thus extending from itchy poison ivy that comprises a personal repetition complex since childhood through the erudite quincunx symbol to the originating point outside both these opposites, a transitional space opens up to meditate upon, to improvise, to pause and play around with the itching and the symbols and the possible meaning coming into view.

The poison ivy body-speech is the slime end of the arc, the primordium from which we all creep and crawl and eventually emerge, and to which we must return for refreshment and regeneration, lest our complexes repeat all our lives. The sophisticated symbols comprise the opposite end of the arc. Here we meet a developed human endeavor, traditions on which we depend, books of symbols written about accumulated human experience, gatherings of insights into the meanings of these symbols. The stone is found between them, constructed and tripped over in the transitional space from which I have been working in this essay, moving around a vexing allergy that has been playing around with me for over half my life. As Jung says, we must look to our greatest problem. There, the creator is experimenting with us.[26] The body kept going after the mystery hiding in the poison ivy, conserving the truth symbolized in the skin's suffering. Healing meant going beyond ego-entanglements with the repeating complex to another level of living and knowing.

If we win through to the stone-hard realization of the meaning of this experience, we will be moved to another mode of existence. Inherited in this event of commonplace poison ivy, neglected when it grows so abundantly by the road, like the ubiquitous *prima materia* from which the *lapis* is fashioned, lie aggregates of human experience that bring us to a new place. Struggling with our problems opens us to an inheritance as abundant as the roadside ivy, and ushers us into the spiritual realm. We are brought *there*. The stone becomes the hard bit of truth, the flint-hard shard of meaning that I can know about directly, that I can carry in my mitten like a favorite blue rock. What is that realm? Where is that truth? Is that spirit to whom we really belong? We cannot define this "other" perhaps, but we can describe its presence. One description that sounds the right note, came from a man, an analysand, who said: "I found myself under regard."

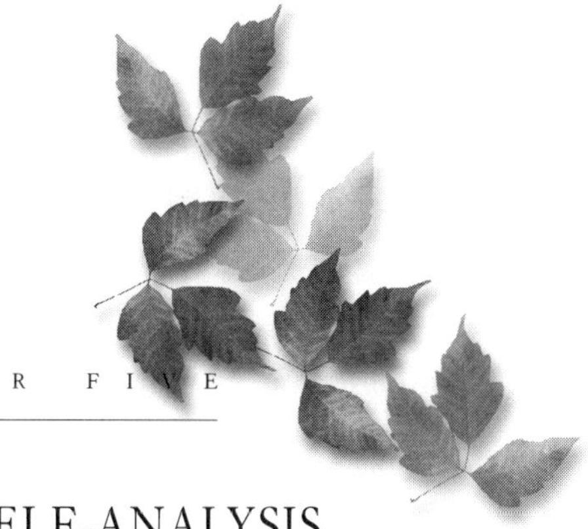

CHAPTER FIVE

A PROJECT *in* SELF-ANALYSIS

"Psychoanalytic inquiry is accustomed to divine secret and concealed things from despised or unnoticed features, from the rubbish heap, as it were, of our observations."[1]

"No theory can eliminate what is the ultimate standard for all theory: that which is given in plain seeing and is, therefore, original."[2]

COMING TO THE END OF THIS PROJECT—NOT JUST the writing of it, but the decade of meditation and internal conversation that led up to the writing—I realize that I have been engaged in a self-analysis. I mean something specific by this: analysis of my self, specifically a part of me that lay dormant for many years, confined to repeating itself within a complex that expressed itself in physical terms. And I mean that this analysis was conducted in relation to the larger Self, in Jung's terms, that superordinate reality that we experience as a ruthless urging going on in us to fill out the space within the boundaries of the particular psychosomatic unity we call our own personal self. With analysands at countless times I have seen that something will not let them go, but insists through incurable symptom, or dogging dream, or restlessness of soul, that they complete themselves, that they come into their own, that they reach all they can be.

Here it was with me now, and with a part of me that stretched all the way from earliest childhood into my sixth decade. Unlike other problems, those that took me into analysis or those I had worked on during analysis, or countertransference problems in my work as an analyst, or just ordinary daily living problems, this poison ivy complex had never been touched, never investigated. It was a neglected problem and it symbolized neglect: what was neglected in my family and where I was neglected. The annual breakout of the noxious poisoning consolidated and expressed this neglect. When the questioning of its meaning burst into consciousness, then it brought with it, like the plant itself with its twining tendrils, not only tangled relations to others but the deepest roots of my own planting-in-being. Poison ivy is notorious for being hard to uproot and eradicate. The roots of this complex, entwined around poison ivy, grew deep into the foundations of my orientation to life, extending out of sight and touch, showing me how I had been positioned in relation to reality, and held fast there.

The questions that kept recurring in this study were: "Held fast for what? Who or what was holding me fast? For what purpose? To what end?" In those questions I discovered that the other partner in this inquiry was the Self, an inner witness or double, a presence that had things to say in response to what my ego was fumbling to formulate. I do not mean to suggest that the Self is ready-made, existing in each of us like another personality. It is not such a clearly given guide, as I have learned in my personal experience and my work as an analyst for over three decades. Its means of manifestation are vastly different from those of the ego. It issues no words or logical constructions, no reasoning arguments to persuade a reluctant ego. No orderly sequence of images set out a clear path for the ego. Instead one meets brute force, such as repetitive poison ivy attacks, or, as clients demonstrate steadily—an intractable insomnia, a felling depression, or fugitive dream fragments that seem cockeyed when looked at in light of day.

For example, when an American analysand is meditating on a feeling of being pressed down by a condensed weight, and asks its origins and its remedy and dreams that night of a Chinese woman inquiring about how to use the comma, we can see how different the conscious and unconscious points of view are. The dreamer asks an urgent question about feeling oppressed, and the dream fishes up a foreigner trying to learn English grammar. In the dream, the dreamer apologizes for not bringing her eyeglasses, which are very tiny, to provide a lens for the elderly Chinese woman to focus with. But the Chinese woman says, no, she does not want glasses; she wants to learn how to use the comma.

It took my analysand and me a while to see that the dream shows the dreamer her usual ego-stance: to focus through the lens of the intellect, to grasp through a concept what the content to be focused upon was (the eye glasses). That way in the dream is shown to be not just missing or forgotten, but tiny. Furthermore, it is not needed or desired. Instead, the way to apprehend is shown in the dream to be through learning the comma's use. A comma is the smallest punctuation mark that allows time for taking a breath, to make a pause. Even in music, the comma represents the minute separation of the flow of notes. The point of view of the Self, speaking through the language of the unconscious, is personified in the dream in an ancient female who lives on the other side, the underside, of the world—the dreamer remembered the childhood game of "digging down to China." The dream shows that comprehension comes through another mode than the intellect's—through breathing, taking a breath, making pauses. Thus the "answer" to the dreamer's meditations is to break up the condensation of weighty self-judgments by first using the smallest means of separation, that of the breath-pause, through the comma. The means of finding the origin and remedy for the pressing weight is minute body-backed breathing, a beginning of differentiation. The dreamer is shown that help comes not from her usual approach, which has always been the intellect moving downward to grasp an answer by means of a focused conceptualizing. Instead, the remedy is found in the breath moving upward through the whole body, bringing *prana*, energy from the center, at first in the smallest possible amounts.

The Self speaks through the language of the unconscious, what Jung called the tumult of chaotic emotions.[3] Intensity of affect pulls one in the right direction. We must submit to a blast of intense emotion and follow it with devotion, not knowing in advance where we are going. This is what Bion means by "tolerating psychic reality." As St. John of the Cross says, a kind of darkness falls because we are required to give up the usual ego-directed thinking that provides a calming orientation. Often no clue emerges to tell us what we are doing or where we are going. Knowing about the process avails little. Instead we move blindly in a second darkness, by intuition, by faith. In the dark, we proceed darkly, groping forward into the unknown by way of unknowing.[4] I have come to appreciate much more the life of the mole and the earthworm. And the mystics comfort me, as examples of those who have gone before into the dark and returned to tell the tale. For, finally, the two darknesses of not knowing where we are going or how we are to do our going, even conceive of it, are capped by a third: the darkness of the one to whom we are proceeding, of discovering what the alchemist Dorn called, the one to whom we belong.

The Goal of Analysis

Doing analysis does not differ much from being in analysis. Analyst or patient—whichever side of the room, whichever chair—both occupy themselves in the venture. Though not in identical ways, both are engaged in hunting a fugitive memory, seeking words for the hard-to-describe symptom, feeling affect building between them, suffering confusion about what exactly is being communicated, feeling buffeted by storms of anger or sorrow, struck silent by endless weeping, held fast by the arrival of insight, moved to awe by a sacred moment of communication, not only between them, but through them and to them from a third presence. When someone consults me for a first interview I always say at the end of the hour that the goal of analysis, as I see it, is to build and maintain a sturdy conversation between yourself and your unconscious, between your conscious sense of self and the psyche living in you. When that is done, you do not need an analyst anymore. The analyst is a translator. When the conversation is ongoing, and you know the language, you can translate for yourself. I am also thinking, but do not usually say aloud, that you will, as well, find yourself translated by this other reality inhabiting you far inside yourself and addressing you from far outside yourself.

Analysis, then, as I see it, is not just problem-fixing; it is a reorientation of attitude and stance toward psychic reality and what communicates itself through it. Using Jung's map, this means that much information and affect come from layers of personal unconscious experience. In addition, bursting through those personal memories come affects and contents that feel larger than our own experiences. The images are primordial, and we feel it to be of the utmost importance to understand and assimilate them into daily living. We feel coming through these deeper patterns a sense of direction, meaning the way to orient our lives toward what matters most. Through this sense of psychic reality comes perception of a larger whole to which we belong. What starts out as a personal quest to solve a problem that shackles us, leads to what or who is standing there as we get unshackled. How do we to live in relation to that?

For me, the ridiculous and painful poison ivy "complex" was a problem to be solved, which revealed itself over time as a conserved state of suffering through which an archaic mind was speaking. Thus I discovered not just the meaning of the complex but also the power of my own subjectivity to find a way to communicate it to me. As Jonathan Lear writes: "A person's subjectivity is powerful not merely because it is striving for expression but also because it may be expressed archaically. Archaic mental functioning knows no firm boundary between mind and body, and so archaic mind is incarnate in the body. Although fantasies may be expressed in images, they may also occur in . . . skin irritations. . . . In this way a person's subjectivity permeates his being." [5]

The poison ivy problem introduced me to layers of subjectivity not under my ego's control. Through those other layers, another "other" was speaking, nudging me this way or that, much as a sheep dog bites the heels of sheep to herd them through narrow gates. It was this "other" I was trying to heed, to see and hear and taste and touch it. It remained present, but elusive. It is truly other, but not absent. That is what I am calling the Self, and what I mean when I say this exercise in self-analysis was under the aegis of the Self.

The goal of analysis is the establishment and maintenance of sturdy conversation between consciousness and the unconscious. Through both, this other Self arrives. Its more personal aspects show forth in our images of its presence and in our experience of an increased subjectivity in ourselves when we converse with it. People call this presence by different names. For Bion, it is 0 and his particular route to it is through thinking. What startles us is how much our images of this "god" include our own problems. Bion's "grid," for example, in my appreciation for his work, includes his schizoid tendencies, which he, himself, describes as such. Bion movingly tells of his inability even to move his body in response to his baby daughter crawling across the floor toward him. He speaks poignantly of his having died in World War I—a death of soul. Serving as a tank commander in the volunteer army, Bion felt himself to be a coward (which he was not, having been awarded the Distinguished Service Order). The shocking loss of one comrade after another seemed to culminate in the death of his friend Asser. In reference to that grief he wrote in his journal, "I died on August 7th on the Amiens-Roye Road." And again, "I never recovered from the *survival* of the Battle of Amiens."[6] When Bion writes of splitting, the reader feels he is speaking not only about his patients but also of himself. These schizoid problems are folded into his arrival at 0 and the way he gets there. This 0 is what lies beyond his schizoid splits, beckoning him toward itself to become one with it, an at-one-ment, which repairs and forgives all that kept him from it. The grid he constructs in clinical sessions maps the route to 0 in the most abstract terms he can find, thus his penchant for geometrical notations and algebraic equations.[7] The ways we block 0 in a clinical session Bion calls our conversation-stopper remarks, which he places in column 2 of his grid.

Bion wants to create a theory that is three-dimensional, like his grid whose vectors proceed both north and south, east and west, stemming from his belief that Euclidean geometry arose originally from attempts to describe the emotional experience of a space once occupied by an object (e.g. the breast) that is no longer there.[8] This two-dimensional grid, whose vectors move in all directions of the compass, also stands forth to map a third vector moving from surface to depth in an actual clinical session by charting how a patient moves from unprocessed thought (beta elements) to thinking (the alpha function) to action (transformation) on the basis of that thinking process. We can see the schizoid tendency to withdraw here translated into a capacity to abstract; the schizoid tendency to observe transformed into the most extreme theoretical generalizations, in order to apply them to as many clinical encounters as possible. Nestled in this attempt to chart how thinking may lead us to avoid or to tolerate psychic reality, is Bion's hope to deliver himself and his patients into experiences of 0.

If Bion stopped here, with only the grid, the schizoid tendencies would dominate his theory. But he does not. He moves and is relentlessly pushed to move on, to "go on going on" as Martin Luther King Jr. says, into 0. This 0 beckons; 0 commands; 0 summons. This 0 is the point of every clinical session, its emotional truth, the point of life. Bion describes it, with his usual clinical acumen, as arriving at being at-one-with 0, but not being 0. To think the latter is maniacal omnipotence, what Jung would call inflation by the mana personality. To be one with 0 fulfills our moving through the three darknesses. Here we arrive at living with truth. We are not the truth, nor do we know about it from a schizoid distance. We live it. Thus 0 for Bion, I believe, conquers and transforms his and our schizoid tendencies by gathering him up into it, which he describes as the ineffable, the ultimate, the godhead. He gets there by thinking, which is both his greatest talent and defense, and he brings this treasure as an offering to what transcends it: 0. Thinking and the grid could be called Bion's God-images, his personal ideas and images for an ultimate mystery that cannot be described.[9]

In Jung's terms, the grid and 0 are Bion's Self-images, that in him which knows about God. Bion's thinking, his grid and his notion of 0, are his subjective God-images, his personal ideas and images for what cannot be described. All this reflects his specific personality, in his historical time and cultural location. His subjective God-images mediate the objective reality that transcends everything, including the psyche. Like Aquinas, who says God is ultimate mystery and our reason breaks down when we try to talk about God because we are trying to talk about what we cannot express and to think about what we cannot think, Bion recognizes that this mystery really exists, but that we cannot know it, we can only live in relation to it. Thus the objective aspect of transcendence exists, but it lies beyond our capacity to apprehend it. Bion's objective God-image, in my terms, is indeed the ultimate mystery.

For Jung, the image of the presence of this other that urges us to complete ourselves is his ambiguous notion of the Self which is and is not God, because, as he says, their images are indistinguishable from each other. His subjective God-image in my terms is the Self, and his route to this presence is through consciousness. The more we are conscious, the more we are conscious both of self and Self. Jung is not unlike St. Augustine, who says that the more we know of ourselves, the more we know of "thee, oh God" and vice versa, *interim te interim me*. Our route can begin with God and end with self, or we can begin with confessions of ourselves and end up with a restlessness that brings us to God. For Jung, at the root of self lies Self. And for Jung, too, accused of psychotic breaks, the steady thrum of consciousness provides the link between the two—the self to the Self and even to what we can call a third—that which transcends the whole psyche.

We experience our personal selves in our particular historical time and cultural space. In his descent to the unconscious Jung said he repeated to himself, "I am a psychiatrist, I live at such and such an address, in such and such a country, I am married and have five children."[10] At those moments, we also experience the incursion of the unconscious—its riotous affects, turbulent emotions, fantastic images, and peculiar logic. If we look at this incoming tide only from the point of view of ego-consciousness reciting its identifying statistics, we will, like Jung, fear we are going mad. But if we can simultaneously entertain the phantasms of unconscious life *alongside* the facts of conscious life, as Jung did, our consciousness will stretch and discover its ground in the unconscious, which shows itself as a medium through which that which transcends the whole psyche communicates to us. From just such a stretching and grounding, Jung found and created his seminal ideas: "The years when I was pursuing my inner images were the most important in my life—in them everything essential was decided . . . the later details are only supplements and clarifications of the material that burst forth from the unconscious, and at first swamped me. It was the *prima materia* for a lifetime's work."[11]

We must understand as well as wonder at the images of the unconscious Jung urges, otherwise we stop much too short of our goal. Our theory is incomplete, then, and worse, says Jung, the unconscious will turn against us in our daily lives. But even understanding is not enough. Understanding must be transformed into ethical action. If we stop at mere wonder and do not proceed to "understanding," negative effects will be conjured up from the unconscious. If we stop at understanding and do not change our behavior, our insight "falls prey to the power principle," which will damage our neighbors as well as ourselves.

We can see in Jung's careful enunciation of the steps of a method of coming to terms with psychic reality—moving from wonder to comprehension to action—that his tendency to become overwhelmed by the unconscious is corrected by careful observation of it and integration of it into living. His personal idiosyncrasies are included in his subjective God-image of the Self. Yet he also believes that he is pointing to an objective reality. He says of the Self that it deconstructs as a symbolic form and that all our personal images for the transcendent finally collapse. Jung says we call the objective reality that transcends us, including the psyche, every kind of name. God puts up with it, and does not defend himself.[12] An objective transcendent reality *does* exist. Jung usually refers to it as God.[13]

Like Bion, who is urged on to living 0, Jung is moved to convert intellectual insight into ethical action. The sequence of image, understanding, and ethical action inscribes on the self allegiance to something well beyond the self and the unconscious. Something new comes through the conjunction of consciousness (meditating on the unconscious) and the unconscious (informing with energy and possibility the conscious viewpoint). We do not know about that something; we live it in transformed behavior: "The images of the unconscious place a great responsibility upon a man. Failure to understand them, or a shirking of ethical responsibility, deprives him of his wholeness and imposes a painful fragmentariness on his life."[14] Like Bion, Jung saw his theory leading into living in a new way. That was its justification: to point to the original which can never be captured in theory, but only enjoyed and endured in the living of it. Arriving at living is what distinguishes a useful and lasting theory from one that fades.

For me, the route to the ineffable, the ultimate infinite godhead, is love—a willingness to seek and find and then receive what is intimated, and then to try to hatch it until something new gets born. Where Jung's dependence on consciousness countered his slipping into psychotic-like episodes, and where Bion's schizoid thinking finally rescued him into a natural living rather than a mere knowing about truth, my need for love and experience of its lack comprised my route to the transcendent. Void, abyss, nothingness vie with a fullness, a vibrant presence.

Each of us brings our particular problems into their solution. Our problems help craft our particular images and understanding of what unfolds as their answer. These images and theories are our subjective God-images. Just as reading Bion gives the impression that he could slide into such extreme schizoid abstractions that one could no longer find him, let alone follow him, reading Jung can deliver one into such a jumble of image, affect, idea that one cannot sort out any clear path.

My own path requires the careful negotiation of huge gaps into which one can plunge as if into a bottomless space. My way of proceeding requires going there into that gap, looking around to see what is there and feeling its reality, even if it is the reality of absence. The stamina required to do that, and the courage, depends on holding fast to love given to and received from others—be they a lover, a friend, a child, an analyst, a beloved pet—a sense of God, a sense of being itself conferred in the design, uniqueness, and bounteous appearance of flowers. The accompanying warmth of feeling allows one to drop into the gap of coldness. As bad as the gap may be, it is finite because we are finite, even in our terrors. Looking for ground that is sure and known to exist brings us human feeling as our guide. The early Christian theologian Origen sounds the right note for me when he says the fall of humanity from grace brought "the chilling loss of the divine 'warmth' of love." In making our way back to God, warmth is restored to the psyche through the warm love given us.[15] This feeling sense which hovers, broods and meditates, receives images that arrive to express what is experienced, and includes reflecting on the experience in thought, and leads to conversation with what presents itself.

For conversation to develop, the ego, that is, we ourselves, must speak up loudly and clearly. The ego position must be enunciated with as much precision and passion as possible. This bringing of our conscious viewpoint, this speaking up, always reflects as well the collective conscious values and thought forms of the culture and historical period in which any of us is embedded. The ego must be as specific as possible for the unconscious to answer in a way that we can grasp. Coming to consciousness about what precisely we do need, or want, or feel, or request, broadens our awareness, forcing us to become cognizant of what is stirring us. Achieving such a mindful position takes a lot of work—brooding, meditating, differentiating the trivial from the essential, the less important from the first thing. We cannot do it lightly or quickly. More often than not, arriving at where we are also means tolerating conflict and anxiety, or some other outsized affect. We must bear the strain, admit the uninvited guest that we would prefer to exclude—the panic, the anger, the depression, the humiliation, the shocking degree of revenge we would seek. Usually, these uninvited affects conflict with our conscious value system, so that allowing them amounts to submitting to the burden of opposites within ourselves. Out of the tension of this push-pull, our question, or cry, or plea addresses itself to the unconscious and to what would communicate to us through the unconscious. Then we wait and receive the first thing that appears.

This conversation is not like a buffet table where we can pick and choose which food we will eat. It is a conversation between two parties, and requires respect for what the "other" says or shows, and a considered careful observation of what the "other" communicates. We must pay attention to what the "other" says, and not think we can exchange it at the table for another choice. We must treat this different perspective as if it issues from a real "other" who is responding to us, or initiating its own point. If we do not understand, and we usually do not at first, time must be taken to reach comprehension. Or, another question, for clarification this time, needs to be asked. It is as if the unconscious partner were like a sentient being to whom we are responding and who we trust to respond to us. The response can be made in any form—an unmistakable body feeling, an image, a memory, a puzzling symbol, a dream, an insightful thought, a creative impulse, a recurrence of a symptom that indicates we have gotten off course. Some analysands hear voices or sounds. Some are moved to dance or put their bodies into specific movements or postures. Some feel an inflooding of soft lambent texture—a kind of peace communicated through touch. Some are greeted by silence, a big enfolding silence. Whatever form the response takes, it puts the ball back into the ego's court and we must reply in turn. And so the conversation goes on.

The conversation of the conscious "I" with the heretofore unconscious content or urge or sentient arrival of something new, informs future action. The conversation leads to action in daily life, to the ethical consequence of what the experience bequeaths. I agree with Bion that "tolerating psychic reality," and with Jung that "confronting the unconscious," that my own "inner conversation," if it is real and to go on as real, must change our way of living. Ethics is not duty; it is overflow. What is bestowed upon us, if received, steps over into concrete living. The incarnation of the new thing that comes into daily living may take time to realize, as this essay illustrates. It took ten years of meditation, and some more years of writing. Part of what makes such sustained attention possible is the ethical overflow. Something flowed into my life that made a remarkable difference—no longer to suffer poison ivy attacks. This freedom wants to be shared with other victims in the Ivy League. Ten years is nothing compared to that liberation!

The contrast between the pitiful poison ivy allergy and the big reality that is granted through it serves to remind us on the one hand how all-too-human our plights and perplexities are, and, on the other hand, that anything can serve to bring us into the presence of reality. That is the generosity of reality. Even the silly single sparrow can live connected up; even a poor single hair on our heads can serve to link us to the source point.

My partner in this venture, this ten-year-long meditation, was not another analyst as it had been earlier in my life with two separate people, for a total of seventeen years. Nor was the partner the experts in other ventures I had made in body-work and yoga postures, nor in the different body activities I engaged in over the years (swimming, manual labor with stones and earth, running, dancing, acupuncture) as the medium of exchange between me and other kinds of consciousness, different from the ego's. As Jung says, "healing comes only from what leads the patient beyond himself and beyond his entanglement in the ego."[16] The partner in this poison ivy project turned out to be what was rising into consciousness and bringing with it an increased capacity in me to receive it. Thus, dreams, associations, uncovered memories, body-speech, states of affect such as sorrow, grief, stark aloneness, as well as rage and arousal, all became a means through which this "other" also made its nearness felt. I felt engineered but not coerced. I felt witnessed while I was struggling to witness what was coming into view.

The Need for Witnessing

All of us depend on someone to mediate the world to us. And, then, we each need to develop our own personal relationship to what is mediated. When a parent dies, or goes crazy, or abandons us, a hole exists in our relation to the world, unless we find others to fill it in. Hans Loewald's basis for believing in the success of analysis is the analyst witnessing to the patient's ego, as the patient revisits and reorganizes relation to her or his past in the present relation to the analyst. The analyst provides new mediation for old events and thus rescues them for present living.[17] This creative repetition corrects repetition compulsion. What makes the difference is that dependency needs are now met, instead of being ignored as in the past, or lost in the exigencies of family troubles, bad schools, or political upheaval.

We need other people to witness our experience all through our lives. This insight provides the basis for Heinz Kohut's formulation of our enduring need for another person's empathic mirroring of us, that allows our narcissistic energies to develop and transform into the precious gifts of humor, wisdom, compassion, empathy, and creativity.[18] Kohut explored at length the pivotal role played by this witnessing self-object in developing our capacity to be a person, just as Winnicott did of what he called the subjective-object, which helps us navigate the transitional space where we find and create our sense of self and symbol.[19] Without these others in our lives, we do not *become* at all; we cease to *be*. The part of me that endured poison ivy did not gain an empathic witness to the pain it caused, nor to the sorrow that underlay it, until I began to look into it myself. I could never be sure of the reality of my suffering until my husband witnessed it, hearing me cry out when lowering myself into the bath. His astonishment that I suffered so much that he found witnessing it unbearable, brought home to me its grave degree. And only after I looked into the poison ivy complex did I myself begin to give witness to the silent sorrow it expressed.

We need an other, an objective object to confirm subjective experience. This was especially true for me because my parents, in their different ways, set examples of isolated stoicism when faced with suffering, rather than witnessing it directly and acknowledging it. My mother rose "above" her suffering, both physical and psychological, and pushed off solicitous concern, then spent long hours in bed doped-up on various medicines. My father did not get sick, and with his car accident did not complain, but just returned to work. My peasant mother merely ate her homemade bread softened in coffee when all her teeth were pulled out, and she never mentioned the whole reordering of her bowels that was required at another time, nor her inability to bear children. Her husband just carried on when he was sick and even in the agonies of war, when he served in the army, never whined about hardship. With peasant energy and courage, all four embodied the philosophy that one works until one drops. One just carries on. I felt shame, then, even contemplating making any fuss at all over something so trivial as poison ivy. I felt mute about my affliction and embarrassed before myself for suffering so much.

The missing witness to my sieges was myself. It was I who never asked what this annual itching frenzy might mean. Only after I looked into the complex surrounding poison ivy did its underlying sorrow become accessible. The process of learning to ask of these other levels of consciousness what they had to say was so slow that I did not seek another analyst and the usual analytical container. No words were available for years, nor any dream images. Only a hovering, listening attentiveness seemed appropriate to what was emerging slowly in the midst of a busy life with family and my work as analyst and professor.

I learned how to witness a recurring experience that had been dissociated from the rest of my life. A conversation began with this lost part of myself. Empathy grew in me for this part of me that suffered from allergies to a plant neglected, at the side of the road, which aptly symbolized what had been neglected in me, as if abandoned by the side of my road. I learned to witness what was unwitnessed. I found, like my husband, it was almost more than I could bear. While I was writing this essay, tumultuous sorrow, grief, and anger rolled in. My skin hurt and sometimes broke out into itching. At one point I felt so ill with fever and flu-like symptoms the doctor thought I had caught Lyme disease, another autoimmune system disorder. When the dreams of poison ivy came, my body was spared, as if shifting its burden into the psychic realm. My own enlarging consciousness slowly gave personal testimony to what poison ivy symbolized for me. In a most personal sense, this was an exercise in lower-case "s" self-analysis.

Yet this project seemed to be sponsored by the Self as well. Under its shelter, it was as if I were the object of its advocacy. The Self as the center of the whole conscious and unconscious psyche seemed to be my witness. Why do I say this? The answer is clear. The conversation began when my ego was searching for meaning, and my dreams tossed up responses at night, and when the symptoms brought in during the day were met by sudden, clear, resounding insights. The previous clanging of colliding opposites slowly transformed into their coincidences and then into their conjunction. As I said earlier, something kept urging me on, nipping at my heels, steering me this way and that. Once I let go of reliance on ego-directed thinking, a synchronous field of energy seem to compose itself around the project. The irrationality of looking for the psychogenic origin of a nonpsychosomatic allergy did not seem to me to be a fool's errand. Or perhaps I was content to be the fool, hanging by my foot upside down in the well, as my dream portrayed me. Upending the ordinary causal way of looking at things led the dream-me to catch sight of the blooming *fleur-de-lis* flower. Its presence changed the bottomless abyss into a well in whose darkness light blossomed.

I knew that some objective meaning existed that connected itself to this poison ivy complex. I was finding it, I was creating it, but it also existed objectively, unfurling toward me, and was not just my subjective creation. My body knew about it more than my mind. Meaning exists in matter too, not just spiritually or psychically. In an idiosyncratic, personal way, through this allergy complex I was being delivered into an order that I was discovering as well as making. Something addressed me, and had repeatedly been addressing me through the annual poison ivy experiences. Once I engaged with this other presence, through all my senses, through all of me, my poison ivy attacks ceased.

I had thought that it was I who was doing the witnessing at long last, no longer neglecting, leaving this split-off part of myself by the side of the road. But I discovered the reverse: something else was witnessing me. My efforts to witness to this cut-off part of my experience were being witnessed. The evidence for this insight was the complete change in matter—my body—when my mind took over the suffering that poison ivy used to inflict on the body. I saw that the unfolding order of meaning spanned both matter and psyche. Order did not arise only from our subjective constructions, which are usually causal, but it arose objectively as well. My looking for the past initiating cause of my poison ivy repetition and for its final future cause—where it was heading, to what purpose—surpassed causality and became grounded in the bigger surroundings of synchronicity. Past causes in my experiences of emotional deprivation proved relevant. Purposes opening into the future supported me in the painful carrying out of this project, but the presence of something more, right in the midst of past and future investigations, enlarged the present into a direct relationship with this presence. That, finally, seemed the point—relationship to this larger presence. That made the pain worth everything, for this living relationship was more important, more alive, than any cause or effect or purpose.

After Analysis, What?

Only in the finishing of this project do I see that it might serve as an example of how any of us who have undertaken analysis, and those of us who do analysis, can envision how to proceed when we are no longer in analysis. How do we go on monitoring cases when finished with classes or supervision? I find myself bringing this up with analysands who are themselves analysts-in-training, about to graduate. Many options are available, but individuals must seek out the one that works for them. More centrally, how will we keep alive the relationship to our unconscious when finished with analysis? How do we go on processing dreams, symptoms, and routine problems when we are no longer in training, or involved in the weekly rounds of analytical treatment? I have been seeing patients since 1962, when I was myself in training. I have been in private practice since 1965, and finished my second training sequence in 1967. I have worked with analysands every year since. How do we keep alive in the same work decade after decade? This is not only a practical and ethical question, but a philosophical and theological one. How do we go on living with what we discovered in analysis about psychic reality and its multiple meanings?

Jung and Bion tell us we cannot name the reality we discover through the psyche, but can only be conscious of it, be consciously related to it, be at one with it. The mystics tell us that their union with the beloved translates into a lavish impulse to serve others in the world in the name of the one they love. The philosopher Paul Ricoeur—whose subjective God-image seems to be the *verbum*, the word which strives to express the inexpressible—writes prolifically. Each translation from his French into English all but buries the reader under an avalanche of words, only to release him to a sudden astonishing *aperçu* that grants glimpses of the reality that lies behind all the words. For me, building a loving connection, a back-and-forth conversation between ego and Self and what lies beyond both, delivers us into living in a new way. The ego, as I said before, must be as specific as possible in its questions and searchings, bringing all our heartfelt concerns and needs into conscious expression in this conversation. Then the responses of the unconscious, and *through* the unconscious, relate to what is sought. It is as if the ego here were the eye of the needle which focuses the All into a relationship to human life lived in the world. For the ego, becoming this focused and clear about what really matters is part of the devotion needed to build this kind of conversation.

An analysand who suffered a difficult beginning in life and a stubborn complex as a result, learned this lesson about specificity anew when landing a much desired and clearly wonderful job. She had spent years feeling, "I'll never be enough." She was adopted in her early years, after being wrenched away in a court battle from a beloved foster mother. But she did not match the fantasy daughter that her adopting mother held dearly, so all through her childhood she felt that she did not "measure up." She was "not enough." She felt that her mother was always mad at her, always berating her with or without words. Now in the face of this new job, her old fears reared up again: she would not be good enough, not what they wanted. She was in danger of staying too general—not considering specifically whether there were aspects of her expertise she needed to develop further in preparation for this new job. She needed to ask concretely, "What do I need to take on to do this new job?" The response from the other side can always answer in reply to the ego question. It may change the question, but we can keep our bearings if we once have a framework in which to receive what comes to us through the unconscious. Otherwise, the unconscious just floods us with its plenty and we simply drown, or float out to sea. If we do not ask anything at all, something defined about what we really do need and desire passionately, then we get no answer, but just drift emptily. Love is passionate and insistent, and keeps spading up what we really desire and what is desired of us, in us.

An End That Is a Beginning

Whatever our route—Bion's thinking, Jung's consciousness, Ricoeur's words, my loving devotion—where do we land? To what do 0, the Self, the *verbum*, the love deliver us? Into *liv-*

ingness. Not into products. Living in touch with what transcends the psyche leads not to products like books, babies, health, wealth, or wisdom. All of those things are important—as is world peace, less killing, protecting the environment, justice for everyone. These are worthy goals all, priceless values. But these are precious by-products only. The main thing is livingness—living in relation to reality, to its origin, to its many sources. Even if we are ill, dying, scarred by long bouts of mental illness, or poor, uncared for in a war-torn country, it is still possible for us to feel the breath of the infinite on our faces, infusing our limbs, something we breathe in and out. How else to explain the simple acts of kindness that continue in the most unspeakable conditions, like concentration camps, or plane crashes? How else to explain the astonishing robustness of spirit in people assaulted by physical handicap, terminal illness, repeated tragedy?

Livingness is living in the reality of what is beyond the psyche, beyond social or physical conditions and constructions, beyond theories and religions. It is living in that reality which somehow, inexplicably, bestows itself upon us. Livingness is living what the alchemists call the *circulatio* of the central energy that moves through all parts of our body, even the lame or missing parts, or the despised ones, feeling that energy flowing into tissue liveness, announcing its pulse, our beat, a zest, conferring on us animated connection to being. We feel glad, happy, fully alive. We touch the spirit by which we live. And the energy flows through all parts of life—other people, the soil, the birds, the grass, even stones and rocks. We feel part of the whole universe. What transcends our goals also infuses them and circulates back and forth between people, with children, at a concert, in the subway.

Etty Hillesum described in letters written from a deportation camp in Nazi-occupied Holland what it felt like to discover the sanctuary of prayer into which she stepped in the midst of screaming babies, frantic mothers, and terrified prisoners—including Etty, her parents, and her brother—waiting to be herded into cattle cars.[20] She stepped out into the cacophony of the camp refreshed and able to look into the eyes of her neighbor, helping however she could, not giving up the reality of the transcendent to the immediate horror of the camp. John of the Cross wrote his love poems to Christ in a prison cell so small he could neither stand nor sit up, and without food on his plate. The ruthlessness of the transcendent consists of the fact that nothing need separate us from it, not even nothingness itself.

The helpfulness of analysis, whether self-analysis or with an analyst, lies in its symbolic discourse. Symbols can point us to what lies beyond them if we believe they point to reality. Symbols cannot be conjured up for convenience sake. We do not get symbols just because we need them or want them. They grow. They convince us by giving us the experience of living contact with what they make available. Symbols are not handy formulas where this stands for that. They include both this *and* that—and more. They bring us to the reality they point to for our living of it, not for simply knowing about it, or for an aesthetic appreciation of it. We live it or we do not live it. If analysis works, it delivers us into this livingness. Symbolic discourse is not the goal. Reality is. After analysis, what? Livingness. It is present even in the neglected roadside poison ivy.

NOTES

Notes to Foreword

1 See Stephen Larsen and Robin Larsen, illus., "The Healing Mask," in *Parabola Magazine: Mask and Metaphor: Role, Imagery, Disguise,* vol. 6, no. 3, August, 1981, p. 78; and Paul Wirz, *Exorcism and the Art of Healing in Ceylon* (Leiden: E. J. Brill, 1954).

Notes to Chapter One: Membership in the Poison Ivy League

1 C. G. Jung, *Letters*, 2 vols. (Princeton: Princeton University Press, 1973/1975), vol. 1, 10 July 1946, pp. 428–429. Brackets mine.

2 See J. and N. Symington, *The Clinical Psychology of Wilfred Bion* (London: Routledge, 1996), pp. 59, 62–63.

3 Bion, W. R. D., *Clinical Seminars and Other Works* (London: Karnac, 1987), p. 248.

4 C. G. Jung, "Concerning Rebirth," *The Archetypes of the Collective Unconscious, Collected Works* vol. 9i (Princeton: Princeton University Press, 1959), §235. Brackets mine. Further references to this title will be to CW9i.

5 C. G. Jung, "The Philosophical Tree," *Alchemical Studies, Collected Works* vol. 13 (Princeton: Princeton University Press, 1967), §397. Further references to this title will be to CW13.

6 Symington, *The Clinical Psychology of Wilfred Bion*, p. 61.

7 Symington, *The Clinical Psychology of Wilfred Bion*, p. 87.

8 C. G. Jung, *The Visions Seminars,* 2 vols. (Zürich: Spring Publications, 1976), vol. 1, p. 30.

9 C. Bollas, *The Shadow of an Object: Psychoanalysis and the Unthought Known* (London: Free Association Books, 1987), pp. 28, 50, 51.

10 C. Bollas, *The Shadow of an Object*, pp. 60–62.

11 C. G. Jung, *Nietzsche's Zarathustra,* 2 vols. (Princeton: Princeton University Press, 1988), vol. 1, p. 196.

12 C. G. Jung, *Nietzsche's Zarathustra,* vol. 1, p. 441.

13 E. Dickinson, *The Complete Poems of Emily Dickinson*, T. H. Johnson, ed. (Boston: Little Brown, 1960), p. 183, No. 384.

14 C. G. Jung, "Instinct and the Unconscious," *The Structure and Dynamics of the Unconscious Collected Works* vol. 8 (Princeton: Princeton University Press, 1960), §270, 275–277, 280. Further references to this title will be to CW8.

15 C. G. Jung, "Synchronicity: An Acausal Connecting Principle," CW8, §967.

16 St. Augustine, *On the Trinity* (Edinburgh: T & T Clark, 1873), p. 357; St. Augustine, *Augustine: Later Works, The Library of Christian Classics* vol. VIII, John Burnaby, ed. (Philadelphia: Westminster Press, 1955), XIII, 12, xi, p. 24.

17 Augustine, *On the Trinity* XI, 24, cited in Burnaby, p.25.

18 Augustine, *On the Trinity* XI, 26–28.

19 Augustine, *On The Trinity* XIV, 18, p. 365.

20 S. W. Jackson, "The Listening Healer in the History of Psychological Healing," *The Journal of Psychiatry* (149:12, December), 1613–1632.

21 C. G. Jung, "Paracelsus as a Spiritual Phenomenon," CW13, §209.

22 C. G. Jung, *Letters* vol. 1, 10 July 1946, p. 429.

23 Since writing this manuscript, which I kept for several years, another attack of poison ivy threatened me on a major holiday weekend after my husband died. I awoke on Sunday, the day before July 4th, with my left eye swelling shut. Had I not been able to secure a prescription for doxycyline, I would have succumbed to a serious siege. I understood this attack as a manifestation of deep grief over the loss of my husband, and, as well, to an additional shock. Someone had stolen my husband's favorite plant from my garden! Being exhausted from nursing my husband in his long day's dying, I had not yet transplanted the large, flowering Oxalis that he loved so much. I simply placed the pot in the garden, thinking I would put it in the ground in a day or two. Then it was gone! My friends thought I was so distraught that I must have forgotten to bring the plant from the city. It was too bizarre, they said, that someone would sneak into my country garden and abscond with the plant. I was frazzled, and doubted my perception. But I knew in my heart a huge theft

had occurred. His death robbed me of a containing love, symbolized even more by the stolen plant. See further notation about this attack in chapter 3, note 6, p. 53.

24 American Academy of Dermatology. "Poison Ivy, Sumac, and Oak" (American Academy of Dermatology, 1999).

25 K. Dōgen, *The Writings of Zen Master Dōgen* (San Francisco Zen Center: North Point Press/Farrar, Straus & Giroux, 1985), pp. 13, 19.

26 K. Dōgen, *The Writings of Zen Master Dōgen*, p. 14.

27 K. Dōgen, *The Writings of Zen Master Dōgen*, pp. 15, 16

28 D. W. Winnicott, "Ego Integration in Child Development," *The Maturational Processes and the Facilitating Environment* (New York: International Universities Press, 1965), pp. 57–58.

29 K. Dōgen, *The Writings of Zen Master Dōgen*, p. 21.

Notes to Chapter Two: A Contact Allergy

1 C. G. Jung, *Two Essays in Analytical Psychology, Collected Works,* vol. 7 (Princeton: Princeton University Press, 1967), §194. Further references will be to CW7.

2 T. L. Tanner, "Rhus (Toxidendron) Dermatitis," *Primary Care* (27, 2, June 2000), p. 498.

3 L. J. Crockett, *Wildly Successful Plants: A Handbook of North American Weeds* (New York: MacMillan, 1977).

4 R. M. Adams, "Dermatitis Caused by Poison Ivy and Its Relatives," *Current Concepts in Skin Disorders* (Spring 1988), pp. 5–9.

5 Adams, "Dermatitis Caused by Poison Ivy and Its Relatives," p. 5; see also, J. Kastner, "Our Country's Plant, Right or Wrong," *New York Times*, November 3, 1991.

6 N. J. Turner and A. S. Szczawinski, *Common Poisonous Plants and Mushrooms of North America* (Portland, OR: Timber Press, 1991), p. 5.

7 American Academy of Dermatology, "Poison Ivy, Sumac, and Oak" (American Academy of Dermatology, 1999) p. 2.

8 Adams, "Dermatitis," p. 7: "Contained in the oil of most of the aforementioned plants is a substance called *urushiol* (from the Japanese word *kiurushi*, meaning sap), a mixture of five catechols containing 15–17 carbon, straight alkyl side chains. The active ingredient is a 3-pentadecacatechol:

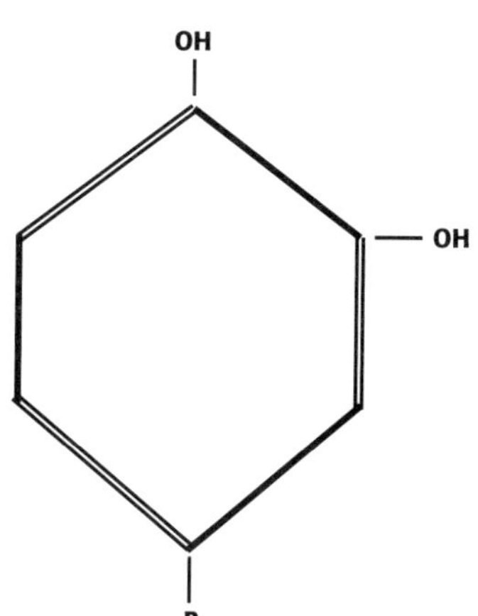

I. $R = (CH_2)_{14}\ CH_3$

II. $R = (CH_2)_7\ CH = CH\ (CH_2)_5\ CH_3$

III. $R = (CH_2)_7\ CH = CHCH_2\ CH + CH\ (CH_2)_5\ CH_3$

IV. $R = (CH_2)_7\ CH = CHCH_2\ CH = CHCH\ = CHCH_3$

V. $R = (CH_2)_7\ CH + CHCH_2\ CH = CHCH_2\ = CH = CH_2$

"The urushiol from *Toxicodendron radicans* (poison ivy), for example, is a mixture of I, II, II, and V. Other plant species vary somewhat in their constituents. The allergenicity of the pentadecacatechol depends upon its degree of unsaturation, the saturated molecules being nearly nonallergenic. Methylation of the hydroxly radicals also renders the molecule nonallergenic. The pentadecacatechols bond covalently with skin protein and evoke a type IV delayed hypersensitivity reaction not only in humans, but also in guinea pigs, mice, and rabbits. The oleoresin is readily released when parts of the plant are crushed or otherwise damaged. Smoke from incompletely burning plants contains particles of the oil, and the heavy sap bonds readily to articles of clothing, tools, animal fur, birds, etc."

9 Turner and Szczawinski, *Common Poisonous Plants*, pp. 21, 88; see also G. Sauer, *Manual of Skin Diseases* (Philadelphia: J. B. Lippincott, 1991) p. 96.

10 S. Moschell and H. Hurley, eds. *Dermatology,* vol. 1 (Philadelphia: W. B. Saunders/Harcourt, Brace, Jovanovitch, 1975), p. 403; see also, *Taber's Cyclopedic Medical Dictionary* (Philadelphia: F. A. Davis Company, 1973), pp. C–143, P–18, V–21.

11 This is the case despite some experiments with hypnosis that indicate that suggestion can block the skin reaction (contagious dermatitis) produced by plants like poison ivy (see T. X. Barber, "Hypnosis, Suggestions, and Psychosomatic Phenomena: A New Look from the Standpoint of

Recent Experimental Studies," *The American Journal of Clinical Hypnosis* (21, 1, July 1978), pp. 13–27.

12 I. Riott, J. Brostoff, D. Male, *Immunology* (Philadelphia: Mosby, 1998), p. 342.

13 T. L. Tanner, "Rhus (Toxicodendron) Dermatitis," p. 497.

14 Riott, *Immunology*, p. 343.

15 Riott, *Immunology*, pp. 342–345; see also G. J. V. Nossal, *Antibodies and Immunity* (New York: Basic Books, 1978), p. 242.

16 A. J. Ziegler, *Archetypal Medicine*, G. V. Hartman, trans.(Woodstock, CT: Spring Publications, 1983), pp. 17, 20.

17 C. G. Jung, *Mysterium Coniunctionis, Collected Works* vol. 14 (Princeton: Princeton University Press, 1970), §14–16, 104–109; see also, C. G. Jung, "Psychology of the Transference" *The Practice of Psychotherapy, Collected Works,* vol. 16 (Princeton: Princeton University Press, 1954), §353–358; see also E. F. Edinger, *Anatomy of the Psyche: Alchemical Symbolism in Psychotherapy* (La Salle, IL: Open Court, 1985), pp. 211–215; see also E. F. Edinger, *The Mystery of the Coniunctio: Alchemical Image of Individuation* (Toronto: Inner City Books, 1994), p. 68; see also E. F. Edinger, *The Mysterium Lectures: A Journey Through C. G. Jung's "Mysterium Coniunctionis"* (Toronto: Inner City Books, 1995), p. 38. Further references to *Collected Works* will be to CW14 and CW16.

18 This phrase is from personal communication of Barry Ulanov.

19 E. F. Edinger, *Mysterium Lectures*, p. 85.

20 A. J. Ziegler, *Archetypal Medicine*, p. 34.

21 D. W. Winnicott, *Playing and Reality* (London: Tavistock, 1971), pp. 2–3.

22 D. W. Winnicott, *Playing and Reality,* chapters 7 and 8.

23 C. G. Jung, *Mysterium Coniunctionis*, §494, 657, 696; see also E. F. Edinger, *Anatomy of the Psyche*, pp. 183–210; see also E. F. Edinger, *The Mystery of the Coniunctio*, pp. 74ff; see also E. F. Edinger, *The Mysterium Lectures*, pp. 38, 85, 279–280, 286, 295.

24 A. J. Ziegler, *Archetypal Medicine*, p. 67.

25 A. B. Ulanov, *Finding Space: Winnicott, God, and Psychic Reality* (Louisville, KY: John Knox/Westminster, 2001), chapter 2.

26 T. Ogden, "On Potential Space," in D. Goldman, *In One's Bones: The Clinical Genius of D. W. Winnicott* (Northvale, NJ: Jason Aronson, 1993), pp. 229–230.

27 C. G. Jung, *Letters,* 2 vols (Princeton: Princeton University Press, 1973 and 1975), vol. 1 p. 429, 10 July 1946.

28 C. G. Jung, "On the Nature of the Psyche," *The Structure and Dynamics of the Psyche, Collected Works,* vol. 8 (Princeton: Princeton University Press, 1969), §406–408. Further references will be to CW8.

29 C. Clément, *The Lives and Legends of Jacques Lacan* (New York: Columbia University Press, 1983), pp. 78, 136.

30 C. Clément, *The Lives and Legends of Jacques Lacan* p. 63.

31 C. Clément, *The Lives and Legends of Jacques Lacan* p. 65,

66; see also, J. Lacan, "Encore," *Seminaire* Book 20 (Paris: Seuil, 1981), pp. 70–71.

32 J.–L. Marion, *Prologoméne à la Charité* (Paris: La Différence, 1986), pp. 146–152, 163–171.

33 H. Beinfield and E. Korngold, *Between Heaven and Earth: A Guide to Chinese Medicine* (New York: Ballantine Books, 1991), pp. 50, 51, 52, 53–54: "The Tao is an undifferentiated whole. It is both the unity of all things and the way the universe works. Out of this oneness emerges *Yin–Yang*: the world in its infinite form. *Yin–Yang* is a symbolic representation of universal process that portrays a changing rather than a static picture of reality. The *Yin–Yang* model is also used to differentiate aspects of the process. Within the magnetic field of fundamental opposition and creative tension, each aspect interrelates, interpenetrates, and depends upon the other. The poles of a unified whole are characterized in relation to each other, revolving cycles of the 'one' becoming the 'other'.... *Yin* is at the core, sinking, condensed, and internal. *Yang* is at the surface, rising, dispersed, and external. . . . *Yang* makes things happen. It transforms. *Yin* provides the material basis for the transforming power of *Yang*. Energy—heat, activity, light—transforms matter. If *Yin* is a noun, then *Yang* is a verb.... Health is defined as the poised balance between *Yin–Yang* disharmony. . . . The internal organs of the body, hidden and protected from external influence, are *Yin* relative to the exposed skin and muscle, which are *Yang*. . . . The exterior surface of human body

(skin, hair, superficial nerves, and blood vessels) is exposed and therefore *Yang*."

34 A. J. Ziegler, *Archetypal Medicine*, p. 68.

35 D. Black, *Allergies: Overreacting to Life* (Springville, UT: The Healing Current Series, 1991), pp. 5–6.

36 D. Black, *Allergies*, p. 6.

37 E. C. Whitmont, *Psyche and Substance* (Berkeley. CA : North Atlantic Books, 1991), p. 139.

38 E. C. Whitmont, *Psyche and Substance*, p. 140.

39 E. C. Whitmont, *Psyche and Substance*, p. 141.

40 E. C. Whitmont, *Psyche and Substance*, p. 142.

41 *Calcarea* and *magnesium* are not used in direct application for allergies. One thinks of them in the "as if" terms of symbols indicating the circulating or blocked flow of life through the two poles of contraction and expansion. (Personal communication with Dr. E. C. Whitmont about these specific pages.)

42 E. C. Whitmont, *Psyche and Substance* pp. 143–144.

Notes to Chapter Three: Personal Dimension

1 C. G. Jung, *The Symbolic Life, Collected Works* vol. 18 (Princeton: Princeton University Press, 1976), §1292. Further references will be to CW18.

2 H. W. Loewald, "On the Therapeutic Action of Psychoanalysis," *Papers on Psychoanalysis* (New Haven, CT: Yale University Press, 1980), p. 242.

3 W. R. Bion, *A Memoir to the Future* (London: Karnac, 1991).

4 C. G. Jung, *Two Essays on Analytical Psychology, Collected Works* vol. 7 (Princeton: Princeton University Press, 1966), §122, 130. Further references will be to CW7.

5 C. G. Jung, CW7, §122, 130

6 There was one small exception, where I caught poison ivy by my own neglect (see chapter 1, p. 19, and note 23). Then there were little flurries of outbreaks when I finally set about to write this manuscript, which I attribute to the stress of what I had uncovered and was trying to describe. As I also relate in chapter 1, note 23 (p. 167), when my husband died and I had lost the container of the life we shared, I awoke one morning to poison ivy having penetrated my left eye. This symbolized to me that my perception was imperiled. The wound to the left side also symbolized to me the piercing of my feminine nature all the way into the unconscious.

7 G. Bright, "Synchronicity as a Basic Analytic Attitude," *Journal of Analytical Psychology* (42, 4, 1997), pp. 613–636.

8 P. Klee, *Pedagogical Sketchbook* (New York: Praeger, 1962), p. 24.

9 C. G. Jung, CW7, §159.

10 C. G. Jung, CW7, §164; see also M. Milner, *On Not Being Able to Paint* (New York: International Universities Press, 1957), pp. 30, 120–121.

11 C. G. Jung, CW7, §164.

12 C. G. Jung, CW7, §184.

13 C. G. Jung, *Nietzsche's Zarathustra* 2 vols. (Princeton: Princeton University Press, 1988), vol. 2, pp. 196, 197.

14 M. Boss, *Psychoanalysis and Daseinanalysis* (New York: Basic Books, 1963), pp. 168–169.

15 D. W. Winnicott, *Human Nature* (London: Free Association Books,1988), p. 42; see also pp. 23, 26, 122; see also D. W. Winnicott, "The Theory of Parent–Infant Relationship," *The Maturational Processes and the Facilitating Environment* (New York: International Universities Press, 1965), pp. 44–45.

16 D. W. Winnicott, "Psycho–Somatic Disorder," *Psychoanalytic Explorations* (London: Karnac. 1964/1969), pp. 103, 115.

17 M. M. R. Khan, *When Spring Comes: Awakenings in Clinical Psychoanalysis* (London: Chatto and Windus, 1988), pp. 18–19.

18 M. M. R. Khan, *When Spring Comes,* p. 24.

19 D. Anzieu, *The Skin Ego: A Psychoanalytic Approach to the Self* (New Haven, CT: Yale University Press, 1989), pp. 4, 9, 13.

20 N. Coltart, *Slouching Towards Bethlehem . . . and Further Psychoanalytic Explorations* (London: Free Association Books, 1992), p. 13.

21 C. Bollas, *The Shadow of an Object: Psychoanalysis and the Unthought Known* (London: Free Association Books, 1987), pp. 59, 134; see also A. Phillips, *Terrors and Experts* (Cambridge, MA: Harvard University Press, 1995), pp. 36–37.

22 H. Johari, *Chakras: Energy Centers of Transformation* (Rochester, VT: Destiny Books, 1987), pp. 65–68.

23 A. Judith, *Eastern Body, Western Mind: Psychology and the Chakra System as a Path to the Self* (Berkeley, CA: Celestial Arts, 1996), p. 59.

24 A. Judith, *Eastern Body, Western Mind.*, pp. 62, 66.

25 C. Myss, *Anatomy of the Spirit* (New York: Three Rivers Press, 1986), pp. 104, 106.

26 C. Myss, *Anatomy of the Spirit* p. 240; see also p. 198.

27 C. Myss, *Anatomy of the Spirit*, p. 202.

28 C. Myss, *Anatomy of the Spirit*, p. 239.

29 C. Myss, *Anatomy of the Spirit*, p. 246; see also p. 249.

30 C. Myss, *Anatomy of the Spirit*, p. 265 (italics mine); See also, Judith, *Eastern Body, Western Mind*, p. 409.

31 J. McDougall, *Theatres of the Body: A Psychoanalytic Approach to Psychosomatic Illness* (London: Free Association Books, 1989), p. 171.

32 D. Anzieu, *The Skin Ego*, p. 17.

33 J. McDougall, *Theatres of the Body*, p. 43.

34 D. W. Winnicott, "The Theory of Parent–Infant Relationship," p. 45; see also D. W. Winnicott, "Ego Integration in Child Development," *The Maturational Processes and the Facilitating Environment* (New York: International Universities Press, 1962/1965), p. 58.

35 J. McDougall, *Theatres of the Body*, p. 28.

36 See pages 18 and 19.

37 A. Ulanov and B. Ulanov, *Religion and the Unconscious* (Louisville, KY: John Knox/ Westminster, 1975), chapter 11.

38 J. E. Circlot, *A Dictionary of Symbols* (New York: Philosophical Library, 1962), pp. 258, 260.

39 J. C. Cooper, *An Illustrated Encyclopedia of Traditional Symbols* (London: Thames & Hudson, 1978/1982), p. 136.

40 D. Anzieu, *The Skin Ego*, pp. 20, 32, 33.

41 A. J. Ziegler, *Archetypal Medicine* (Woodstock, CT: Spring Publications, 1983), p. 64.

42 D. Anzieu, *The Skin Ego*, p. 34n; see also p. 201.

43 J. McDougall, *Theatres of the Body*, p. 54.

44 C. G. Jung, *Mysterium Coniunctionis, Collected Works* vol. 14 (Princeton: Princeton University Press, 1963), §193. Further references will be to CW14.

45 C. G. Jung, *Psychology and Alchemy, Collected Works* vol. 12 (Princeton: Princeton University Press, 1968), §94. Further references will be to CW12.

46 M. M. R. Khan, *Alienation in Perversions* (New York: International Universities Press, 1979), p. 54.

47 M.-L. von Franz, *Alchemy: An Introduction to the Symbolism and the Psychology* (Toronto: Inner City Books, 1959/1980), p. 103; see also M.-L. von Franz, *The Psychological Meaning of Redemption Motifs in Fairy Tales* (Toronto: Inner City Books, 1956/1980), pp. 23–25, 28–30; see also A. J. Ziegler, *Archetypal Medicine*, p. 69.

48 H. Searles, "Positive Feelings in the Relationship Between the Schizophrenic and His Mother," *Collected Papers on Schizophrenia and Related Subjects* (New York: International Universities Press, 1965), p. 220.

49 C. G. Jung, CW14, §336, n. 662.

50 E. F. Edinger, *Anatomy of the Psyche: Alchemical Symbolism in Psychotherapy* (La Salle, IL: Open Court, 1985), p. 76.

51 E. F. Edinger, *Anatomy of the Psyche,* p. 58.

52 P. Dale–Green, "The Symbolism of the Toad," *The Guild of Pastoral Psychology* (Guild Lecture, 10 July, 1960), p. 14.

53 P. Dale–Green, "The Symbolism of the Toad," p. 14.

54 This, and the next two references, are from P. Dale–Green, "The Symbolism of the Toad," p. 15.

55 P. Dale–Green, "The Symbolism of the Toad," p. 16.

56 P. Dale–Green, "The Symbolism of the Toad," p. 16.

57 P. Dale–Green, "The Symbolism of the Toad," p. 18.

58 J. C. Cooper, *An Illustrated Encyclopedia of Traditional Symbols*, p. 157.

59 E. Neumann, *The Great Mother: An Analysis of the Archetype* (Princeton: Princeton University Press, 1955), pp. 194–195.

60 K. T. Preuss, *Die Eingeborenen Amerikas*, Alfred Bertholet, ed. Religiongeschictliches Lesebuch, No. 2, p. 44, cited in Neumann, *The Great Mother*, p. 194.

61 E. Neumann, *The Great Mother*, p. 194.

62 E. Y. Siegelman, *Metaphor and Meaning in Psychotherapy* (New York; Guilford Press, 1990), pp. 3–4, 43–44. 164–165.

Notes to Chapter Four: Archetypal Dimension

1 C. G. Jung, "The Tavistock Lectures" *The Symbolic Life, Collected Works,* vol. 18 (Princeton: Princeton University Press, 1976), §231.

2 R. A. Lockhart, *Psyche Speaks* (New York: Barker Foundation and C. G. Jung Foundation for Analytical Psychology, 1982).

3 C. G. Jung, "The Secret of the Golden Flower," *Alchemical Studies, Collected Works,* vol. 13 (Princeton: Princeton University Press, 1968), §55.

4 C. G. Jung, *Letters,* 2 vols. (Princeton: Princeton University Press, 1973/1975), vol. 1, 1 October 1953, p. 130.

5 C. G. Jung, *Psychological Types, Collected Works,* vol. 6 (Princeton: Princeton University Press, 1971), §426.

6 C. G. Jung, "Spirit and Life," *The Structure and Dynamics of the Psyche, Collected Works,* vol. 8 (Princeton: Princeton University Press, 1969), §644.

7 C. G. Jung, *Dream Analysis* (Princeton: Princeton University Press, 1984), p. 330; see also A. B. Ulanov, "Jung and Prayer," in *Religion and Spirituality in Carl Jung* (Mahwah, NJ: Paulist Press, 1999).

8 R. Kradin, "The Psychosomatic Symptom and the Self: A Siren's Song," *Journal of Analytical Psychology* (42, 3), pp. 405–424.

9 C. G. Jung, *Nietzsche's Zarathustra,* 2 vols. (Princeton: Princeton University Press, 1988), vol. 2, p. 432.

10 D. Anzieu, *The Skin Ego: A Psychoanalytic Approach to the Self* (New Haven, CT: Yale University Press), pp. 50ff.

11 J.-L. Marion, *Prologomène à la Charité* (Paris: La Différence, 1986), pp. 19f.

12 R. A. Lockhart, *Psyche Speaks*, pp. 48–49.

13 C. G. Jung, *Mysterium Coniunctionis*, *Collected Works*, vol. 14, §40–41; E. F. Edinger, *The Mysterium Lectures, A Journey Through C. G. Jung's Mysterium Coniunctionis* (Toronto: Inner City Books, 1995), pp. 57–58; E. F. Edinger, *The Aion Lectures: Exploring the Self in C. G. Jung's "Aion"* (Toronto: Inner City Books, 1996), p. 160.

14 C. G. Jung, *Aion: Researches into the Phenomenology of the Self, Collected Works* vol. 9i (Princeton: Princeton University Press, 1959) §255; E. F. Edinger, *The Aion Lectures*, p. 131; see also C. G. Jung, CW14, §42–50.

15 M. Lurker, *An Illustrated Dictionary of the Gods and Symbols of Ancient Egypt* (London: Thames & Hudson, 1974/1992), pp. 58–59.

16 A. B. Ulanov, *The Wizard's Gate: Picturing Consciousness* (Einsiedeln, Switzerland: Daimon, 1994).

17 A. E. Waite, *The Pictorial Key to the Tarot* (York Beach, ME: Samuel Weiser, 1973), p. 119; K. D. Newman, *The Tarot: A Myth of Male Initiation* (New York: A Quadrant Monograph, C. G. Jung Foundation, 1983), pp. 55–57.

18 J. C. Cooper, *An Illustrated Encyclopedia of Traditional Symbols* (London: Thames & Hudson), 1982), p. 69.

19 B. Matthews, trans., *The Herder Dictionary of Symbols* (Wilmette, IL: Chiron, 1993), p. 78.

20 C. G. Jung, CW9i, §252; E. F. Edinger, *The Aion Lectures*, p. 130.

21 C. G. Jung, CW9i, §252.

22 C. G. Jung, *Nietszche's Zarathustra*, vol. 1, p. 64.

23 Barry Ulanov, personal communication.

24 C. G. Jung, *Memories, Dreams, Reflections* (New York: Pantheon, 1963), p. 21.

25 A. O. Howell, *The Dove in the Stone, Finding the Sacred in the Commonplace* (Wheaton, IL: Quest Books, 1988), pp. 15–26.

26 C. G. Jung, *Letters*, vol. 1 9, September, 1948, p. 509.

Chapter Five: A Project in Self–Analysis

1 S. Freud, "The Moses of Michelangelo," *Standard Edition,* vol. XIII (London: Hogarth Press, 1973), pp. 211–238.

2 E. Husserl, *Introduction to the Logical Investigations: A Draft of a Preface to the Logical Investigations* (the Hague, 1975) in P. J. McCormick, *Modernity, Aesthetics and the Bounds of Art* (Ithaca: Cornell University Press, 1990).

3 C. G. Jung, *Memories, Dreams, Reflections* (New York: Pantheon, 1963), p. 177.

4 John of the Cross, *Ascent of Mount Carmel: The Complete Works of St. John of the Cross* 3 vols. (Westminster, MD: Newman Press, 1953), pp. 17–21, 214; W. R. Bion, *Transformations* (London: Maresfield Library, 1991), pp. 158–159; A. B. Ulanov, "The Holding Self: Jung and the Desire of Being," 1992, in *Religion and Spirituality in Carl Jung* (Mahwah, NJ: Paulist Press, 1999) and in F. R. Halligan and J. J. Shea, eds., *The Fires of Desire: Erotic Energies and the Spiritual Quest* (New York: Crossroad, 1992), pp. 146–170.

5 J. Lear, *Love and Its Place in Nature* (New York: Farrar, Straus & Giroux, 1990), p. 37.

6 Cited in J. S. Grotstein's review of W. R. Bion, *War Memories 1917–1919*, in *Journal of Analytical Psychology*, 1998, vol. 43, no. 4, pp. 610–614.

7 W. R. Bion, *Transformations*, pp. 93, 101, 108, 133–135, 145, 163.

8 W. R. Bion, *Transformations,* pp. 124–125.

9 For more discussion of God–images, see A. B. Ulanov, *Finding Space: Winnicott, God, and Psychic Reality* (Louisville, KY: John Knox/Westminster, 2001), chapter 2.

10 See C. G. Jung, *Memories, Dreams, Reflections*, pp. 181, 189.

11 See C. G. Jung, *Memories, Dreams, Reflections*, p. 199.

12 C. G. Jung, *Nietzsche's Zarathustra,* 2 vols. (Princeton: Princeton University Press, 1988), vol. 1, p. 39.

13 See C. G. Jung, *Memories, Dreams, Reflections*, p. 325.

14 C. G. Jung, *Memories, Dreams, Reflections,* p. 193.

15 B. Drewery, "Deification" in *Christian Spirituality*: *Essays in Honour of Gordon Rupp* ed. Peter Brooks (London: SCM Press, 1975),pp. 33–62.

16 C. G. Jung, "The Philosophical Tree," *Alchemical Studies, Collected Works,* vol. 13 (Princeton: Princeton University Press, 1968), §397.

17 H. W. Loewald, "On the Therapeutic Action of Psychoanalysis," *Papers on Psychoanalysis* (New Haven, CT: Yale University Press, 1980), pp. 225, 230, 241; H. W. Loewald, "Some Considerations of Repetition and Repetition Com-

pulsion," *Papers on Psychoanalysis* (New Haven, CT: Yale University Press, 1980), p. 93.

18 H. Kohut, *The Analysis of the Self* (Chicago: Chicago University Press, 1971), pp. 324ff.

19 D. W. Winnicott, *Playing and Reality* (London: Tavistock, 1971), chapters 1, 3, 4.

20 E. Hillesum, *An Interrupted Life: The Diaries of Etty Hillesum* (New York: Pantheon, 1983); see also, E. Hillesum, *Letters from Westerbork* (New York: Pantheon, 1986).

BIBLIOGRAPHY

I warmly thank the analysands who gave me permission to use their material.

Adams, R. M. "Dermatitis Caused by Poison Ivy and Its Relatives," *Current Concepts in Skin Disorders*. Spring, 1988.

Alexander, F. *Psychosomatic Medicine*. New York: Norton, 1950.

American Academy of Dermatology. "Poison Ivy, Sumac, and Oak." American Academy of Dermatology, 1999.

Anzieu, D. *The Skin Ego: A Psychoanalytic Approach to the Self*. Chris Turner, trans. New Haven: Yale University Press, 1989.

———, ed. *Psychic Envelopes*. London: Karnac, 1990.

Arnold, H., R. Odom, W. James. "The Sensitising Capacity Related to the Capacity to Link with Proteins." *Andrews' Diseases of the Skin: Clinical Dermatology*, 8th edition. Philadelphia: W. B. Saunders Co./Harcourt, Brace, Jovanovitch, 1990.

Augustine, St. *On the Trinity*. Arthur West Hadden, trans. Edinburgh: T &T Clark, 1873.

———. *Augustine: Later Works.* John Burnaby, ed. *The Library of Christian Classics*, vol. VIII. Philadelphia: Westminster Press, 1955.

Barber, T. X. "Hypnosis, Suggestions, and Psychosomatic Phenomena: A New Look from the Standpoint of Recent Experimental Studies." *The American Journal of Clinical Hypnosis*, 21, July, 1978.

Baumgardt, J. P. "Poisonous Plants." *American Horticulture*. 51:26–30, n.d.

Beinfield, H. and E. Korngold. *Between Heaven and Earth: A Guide to Chinese Medicine*. New York: Ballantine Books, 1991.

Bick, E. "The Experience of the Skin in Early Object-Relations." *The International Journal of Psycho-Analysis*, 49, 1968.

Bion, W. R. D. *Attention and Interpretation*. London: Tavistock, 1970.

———. *Clinical Seminars and Other Works*. Francesca Bion, ed. London: Karnac, 1987.

———. *A Memoir to the Future*. London: Karnac, 1991.

———. *Transformations*. London: Maresfield Library, 1991.

———. *War Memoirs 1917–1919*. Francesca Bion, ed. London: Karnac, 1997.

Black, D. *Allergies: Overreacting to Life*. Springville, UT: The Healing Current Series, 1991.

Bollas, C. *Being a Character*. New York: Hill and Wang, 1992.

———. *The Shadow of an Object: Psychoanalysis and the*

Unthought Known. London: Free Association Books, 1987.

Boss, M. *Psychoanalysis and Daseinanalysis*. Ludwig B. Lefebre, trans. New York: Basic Books, 1963.

Bright, G. "Synchronicity as a Basic Analytical Guide," *Journal of Analytical Psychology*, 42, 4, 1997.

Circlot, J. E. *A Dictionary of Symbols*. Jack Sage, trans. New York: Philosophical Library, 1962.

Clark, G. "The Animating Body: Psychoid Substance as a Mutual Experience of Psychosomatic Disorder. *The Journal of Analytical Psychology*, 41, 3, July, 1996.

Clément, C. *The Lives and Legends of Jacques Lacan*. Arthur Goldhammer, trans. New York: Columbia University Press, 1983.

Coltart, N. *Slouching Towards Bethlehem . . . and Further Psychoanalytic Explorations*. London: Free Association Books, 1992.

Cooper, J. C. *An Illustrated Encyclopedia of Traditional Symbols*. London: Thames & Hudson, 1978/1982.

Crockett, L. J. *Wildly Successful Plants: A Handbook of North American Weeds*. New York: MacMillan, 1977.

Dale-Green, P. "The Symbolism of the Toad." Guild Lecture 10, July, 1960. London: The Guild of Pastoral Psychology.

Deutsch, F. *On the Mysterious Leap from the Mind to the Body*. New York: International Universities Press, 1959.

Dickinson, E. *The Complete Poems of Emily Dickinson*. Boston: Little Brown, 1960.

Dōgen, K. *The Writings of Zen Master Dōgen*. Kazuaki Tanahashi, ed. San Francisco: North Point Press, Farrar/Straus & Giroux, 1985.

Doughtery, N., and J. West. "Skin Boundaries, Penetrations, and Power." Chicago: National Meeting of Jungian Analysts, 1997.

Drewery, B. "Deification," in *Christian Spirituality: Essays in Honour of Gordon Rupp*. P. Brooks, ed. London: SCM Press, 1975

Dunbar, F. *Mind and Body: Psychosomatic Medicine*. New York: Random House, 1947.

Dunne, C. "The Roots of Memory." *Spring*, 1988.

Edinger, E. F. *The Aion Lectures: Exploring the Self in C. G. Jung's "Aion*." Deborah A. Wesley, ed. Toronto: Inner City Books, 1996.

———. *Anatomy of the Psyche: Alchemical Symbolism in Psychotherapy*. La Salle, IL: Open Court, 1985.

———. *The Mysterium Lectures: A Journey Through C. G. Jung's "Mysterium Coniunctionis*." Joan Dexter Blackmer, ed. Toronto: Inner City Books, 1995.

———. *The Mystery of the Coniunctio: Alchemical Image of Individuation*. Joan Dexter Blackmer, ed. Toronto: Inner City Books, 1994.

Freud, S. "The Moses of Michelangelo." *Standard Edition,* vol. XIII, London: Hogarth Press, 1973.

Gillespie, R. D. "Psychological Aspects of Skin Disease." *The British Journal of Dermatology*, 50, 1, 1938.

Grotstein, J. S. Review of Bion, W. R. *War Memories 1917–1919. Journal of Analytical Psychology*, vol. 43, no. 4, 1998.

Hill, E. W. and P. M. Mullen. "An Overview of Psychoimmunology: Implications for Pastoral Care." *The Journal of Pastoral Care*, 50, 3, Fall, 1996.

Hillesum, E. *An Interrupted Life: The Diaries of Etty Hillesum*. A. J. Pomerans, trans. New York: Pantheon, 1986.

———. *Letters from Westerbork*. A. J. Pomerans, trans. New York: Pantheon, 1986.

Howell, A. O. *The Dove in the Stone: Finding the Sacred in the Commonplace*. Wheaton, IL: Quest Books/Theosophical Publishing House, 1988.

Husserl, E. *Introduction to the Logical Investigations: A Draft of a Preface to the Logical Investigations*. P. J. Bossert and C. H. Peters, trans. The Hague, 1975, quoted in P. J. McCormick, *Modernity, Aesthetics, and the Bounds of Art*. Ithaca: Cornell University Press, 1913/1990.

Jackson, S. W. "The Listening Healer in the History of Psychological Healing." *The Journal of Psychiatry*, 149:12, December, 1992.

Johari, H. *Chakras: Energy Centers of Transformation*. Rochester, VT: Destiny Books, 1987.

John, St. of the Cross. *Ascent of Mount Carmel*, in *The Complete Works of St. John of the Cross*, vol. I of III. E. Allison Peers, ed. and trans. Westminster, MD: The Newman Press, 1953.

Judith, A. *Eastern Body, Western Mind: Psychology and the*

Chakra System as a Path to the Self. Berkeley, CA: Celestial Arts, 1996.

Jung, C. G. *Aion: Researches into the Phenomenology of the Self. Collected Works*, vol. 9i. Bollingen Series XX, R. F. C. Hull, trans. Princeton: Princeton University Press, 1959.

———. "Paracelsus as a Spiritual Phenomenon," 1942. *Alchemical Studies. Collected Works*, vol. 13. Bollingen Series XX, R. F. C. Hull, trans. Princeton: Princeton University Press, 1968.

———. "The Philosophical Tree," 1945. *Alchemical Studies. Collected Works*, vol. 13. Bollingen Series XX, R. F. C. Hull, trans. Princeton: Princeton University Press, 1968.

———. "The Secret of the Golden Flower," 1929. *Alchemical Studies. Collected Works*, vol. 13. Bollingen Series XX, R. F. C. Hull, trans. Princeton: Princeton University Press, 1968.

———. "Concerning Rebirth," 1939. *The Archetypes of the Collective Unconscious. Collected Works,* vol. 9i, Bollingen Series XX, R. F. C. Hull, trans. Princeton: Princeton University Press, 1959.

———. *Dream Analysis*. Bollingen Series XCIX-1. Princeton: Princeton University Press, 1984

———. *Letters*, 2 vols., Bollingen Series No. 95, Gerhard Adler and Aniela Jaffé, eds. R. F. C. Hull, trans. Princeton: Princeton University Press, 1973/1975.

———. *Memories, Dreams, Reflections*. Aniela Jaffé, ed.

Richard and Clara Winston, trans. New York: Pantheon, 1963.

———. *Mysterium Coniunctionis. Collected Works*, vol. 14. Bollingen Series XX, R. F. C. Hull, trans. Princeton: Princeton University Press, 1970.

———. *Nietzsche's Zarathustra*. 2 vols. Bollingen Series XCIX, James L. Jarrett, ed. Princeton: Princeton University Press, 1988.

———. "Psychology of the Transference," 1946. *The Practice of Psychotherapy. Collected Works,* vol. 16, Bollingen Series XX, R. F. C. Hull, trans. Princeton: Princeton University Press, 1954.

———. *Psychological Types. Collected Works,* vol. 6, Bollingen Series XX, R. F. C. Hull, trans. Princeton: Princeton University Press, 1971.

———. *Psychology & Alchemy. Collected Works*, vol. 12 Bollingen Series XX, R. F. C. Hull, trans. Princeton: Princeton University Press, 1968.

———. "Instinct and the Unconscious," 1919. *The Structure and Dynamics of the Unconscious, Collected Works*, vol. 8. Bollingen Series XX, R. F. C. Hull, trans. Princeton: Princeton University Press, 1969.

———. "On the Nature of the Psyche," 1947. *The Structure and Dynamics of the Unconscious, Collected Works*, vol. 8. Bollingen Series XX, R. F. C. Hull, trans. Princeton: Princeton University Press, 1969.

———. "Spirit and Life," 1919. *The Structure and Dynamics of the Unconscious*, *Collected Works*, vol. 8. Bollingen Series XX, R. F. C. Hull, trans. Princeton: Princeton University Press, 1969.

———. "Synchronicity: An Acausal Connecting Principle," 1952. *The Structure and Dynamics of the Unconscious*, *Collected Works*, vol. 8. Bollingen Series XX, R. F. C. Hull, trans. Princeton: Princeton University Press, 1969.

———. "The Tavistock Lectures," 1935. *The Symbolic Life*. *Collected Works,* vol. 18, Bollingen Series XX, R. F. C. Hull, trans. Princeton: Princeton University Press, 1976.

———. *Two Essays on Analytical Psychology*. *Collected Works*, vol. 7. Bollingen Series XX, R. F. C. Hull, trans. Princeton: Princeton University Press, 1966.

———. *The Visions Seminars*. 2 vols. Zürich: Spring Publications, 1976.

Kastner, J. "Our Country's Plant, Right or Wrong." *New York Times*, November 3, 1991.

Khan, M. M. R. *Alienation in Perversions*. New York: International Universities Press, 1979.

———. *When Spring Comes; Awakenings in Clinical Psychoanalysis*. London: Chatto and Windus, 1988.

Klander, J. V. "Psychogenic Aspects of Skin Disease." *Archives of Neurology and Psychiatry*, 33, 1935.

Klee, P. *Pedagogical Sketchbook*. Sibyl Moholy-Nagy, trans. New York: Praeger, 1925/1962.

Kohut, H. *The Analysis of Self.* Chicago: Chicago University Press, 1971.

Kradin, R. "The Psychosomatic Symptom and the Self: A Sirens' Song." *The Journal of Analytical Psychology*, 42, 3, 1997.

Lacan, J. "Encore" *Seminaire*. Book 20. Paris: Seuil, 1981.

Lear, J. *Love and Its Place in Nature*. New York: Farrar, Straus & Giroux, 1990.

Lief, H., V. Lief, and N. Lief, *The Psychological Basis of Medical Practice*. New York: Harper & Row, 1969.

Lockhart, R. A. *Psyche Speaks*. The Inaugural Series of the C. G. Jung Lectures. New York: Barker Foundation and C. G. Jung Foundation for Analytical Psychology, 1982.

Loewald, H. W. "On the Therapeutic Action of Psychoanalysis," 1957. *Papers on Psychoanalysis*. New Haven, CT.: Yale University Press, 1980.

———. "Some Considerations of Repetition and Repetition Compulsion," 1965. *Papers on Psychoanalysis*. New Haven: Yale University Press, 1980.

Lurker, M. An Illustrated Dictionary of Gods and Symbols of Ancient Egypt. London: Thames & Hudson, 1974/ 1992.

McDougall, J. *The Many Faces of Eros*. New York: Norton, 1995.

———. *Theatres of the Body: A Psychoanalytic Approach to Psychosomatic Illness*. London: Free Association Books, 1989.

McGuire, A. "The Relationship Between the Unconscious Psyche and the Organ of the Skin." *Harvest*. 18, 1972.

Marion, J-L. *Prologemène à la Charité*. Paris: La Différence, 1986.

Maslach, C., G. Marshall, and P. Zimbardo. "Hypnotic Control of Peripheral Skin Temperature: A Case Report." *Psychophysiology*, 9, 6, 1972.

Matthews, Boris. trans., *The Herder Dictionary of Symbols.* Wilmette, IL: Chiron, 1993.

Milner, M. *On Not Being Able to Paint*. New York: International Universities Press, 1957.

Moschell, S. and H. Hurley. *Dermatology*, vol. 1, 3rd ed. Philadelphia: W. B. Saunders/Harcourt, Brace, Jovanovitch, 1975.

Myss, C. *Anatomy of the Spirit*. New York: Three Rivers Press, 1986.

Nathan, T. "Two Dream Representations of the Ego-Skin." D. Anzieu. ed. *Psychic Envelopes*. London: Karnac, 1990.

Neumann, E. *The Great Mother: An Analysis of the Archetype*. Princeton: Princeton University Press, 1955.

Newman, K. D. *The Tarot: A Myth of Male Initiation*. New York: Quadrant Monograph/C. G. Jung Foundation, 1983.

Nossal, G. J. V. *Antibodies and Immunity*. New York: Basic Books, 1978.

Ogden, T. "On Potential Space." Dodi Goldman, ed. *In One's Bones: The Clinical Genius of Winnicott*. Northvale, NJ: Jason Aronson, 1993.

O'Kane, F. *Sacred Chaos: Reflections on God's Shadow and the Dark Self*. Toronto: Inner City Books, 1994.

Phillips, A. *Terrors and Experts.* Cambridge, MA: Harvard University Press, 1995.

Preuss, K. T. *Die Eingeborenen Amerikas: Religionsgeschichtliches Lesebuch*, No. 2. Alfred Bertholet, ed. Tübingen, 1926.

Riott, I., J. Brostoff, and D. Male. *Immunology*. Philadelphia: Mosby, 1998.

Sauer, G. *Manual of Skin Diseases*. Philadelphia: J. B. Lippincott, 1991.

Searles, H. "Positive Feelings in the Relationship Between the Schizophrenic and His Mother," 1958. *Collected Papers on Schizophrenia and Related Subjects*. New York: International Universities Press, 1965.

Schwartz-Salant, N. and M. Stein, eds. *Liminality and Transitional Phenomena*. Wilmette, IL: Chiron, 1991.

Siegelman, E. Y. *Metaphor and Meaning in Psychotherapy*. New York: Guilford Press, 1990.

Sutherland, J. D. *Fairbairn's Journey into the Interior*. London: Free Association Books, 1989.

Symington, J. and N. *The Clinical Psychology of Wilfred Bion*. London: Routledge, 1996.

———. Lecture on Bion. New York Association for Analytical Psychology. New York: January, 1996.

Taber. *Taber's Cyclopedic Medical Dictionary*. Philadelphia: F. A. Davis, 1973.

Tanner, T. L. "Rhus (Toxidendron) Dermatitis," *Primary Care*, June, 2000.

Turner, N. J. and A. S. Szczawinski, *Common Poisonous Plants and Mushrooms of North America*. Portland, OR: Timber Press, 1991.

Ulanov, A. B. *Finding Space: Winnicott, God, and Psychic Reality*. Louisville, KY: John Knox/Westminster, 2001.

———. "The Holding Self: Jung and the Desire of Being." *Religion and Spirituality in Carl Jung*. Mahwah, NJ: Paulist Press, 1999. Also in *The Fires of Desire, Erotic Energies and the Spiritual Quest*. Frerica R. Halligan and John J. Shea, eds. New York: Crossroad, 1992.

———. "Jung and Prayer." *Religion and Spirituality in Carl Jung*. Mahwah, NJ: Paulist Press, 1999. Also in *Jung and the Monotheisms*. Joel Ryce-Menuhin, ed. London: Routledge, 1994.

———. *The Wizards' Gate: Picturing Consciousness*. Einsieddn, Switzerland: Daimon Verlag, 1994.

Ulanov, A. B. and B. Ulanov. *Religion and the Unconscious*. Louisville, KY: John Knox/Westminster, 1975.

von Franz, M-L. *The Psychological Meaning of Redemption Motifs in Fairy Tales*. Toronto: Inner City Books, 1956/1980.

———. *Alchemy: An Introduction to the Symbolism and the Psychology*. Toronto: Inner City Books, 1959/1980.

Wachtel, C. *The Psycho-Medical Guide*. New York: The Psycho-Medical Library, 1956.

Waite, A. E. *The Pictorial Key to the Tarot*. York Beach, ME: Samuel Weiser, 1973.

Weatherhead, L. *Psychology, Religion, and Healing*. London: Hodder & Stoughton, 1952.

Weiss, E. *Psychosomatic Medicine*. Philadelphia: W. B. Saunders, 1957.

Whitmont, E. C. *Psyche and Substance*. Berkeley: North Atlantic Books, 1991.

Winnicott, D. W. *The Child, the Family and the Outside World*. London: Penguin Books, 1964/1975.

———. *Holding and Interpretation: Fragment of an Analysis*. New York: Grove Press, 1986.

———. *Human Nature*. London: Free Association Books, 1988.

———. "Ego Integration in Child Development," 1962. *The Maturational Processes and the Facilitating Environment*. New York: International Universities Press, 1965.

———. "The Theory of the Parent-Infant Relationship," 1960. *The Maturational Processes and the Facilitating Environment*. New York: International Universities Press, 1965.

———. *Playing and Reality*. London: Tavistock, 1971.

———."Psycho-Somatic Disorder," 1964. *Psychoanalytic Explorations*. Clare Winnicott, Ray Shepherd, Madeleine Davis, eds. London: Karnac, 1989.

———. "Mind and Its Relation to the Psyche-Soma," 1949. Winnicott, D. W. *Through Paediatrics to Psycho-Analysis*. New York: Basic Books, 1975.

Ziegler, A. J. *Archetypal Medicine,* G. V. Hartman, trans. Woodstock, CT: Spring Publication, 1983.

INDEX

Index

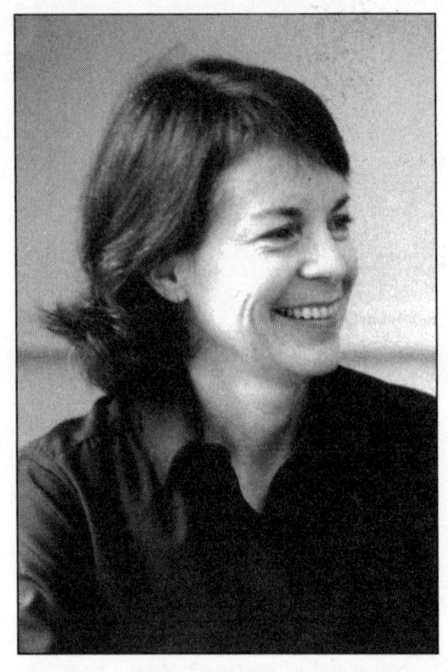

ANN BELFORD ULANOV is a well known and respected Jungian analyst who is active in both Jungian and theological circles. She has written many book over the years—by herself and with her husband, Barry, including *Wisdom of the Psyche*, *The Healing Imagination*, *Religion and the Spiritual in Carl Jung*. She has been an analyst for over thirty-five years. She is a psychoanalyst in private practice, the Christiane Brooks Johnson Professor of Psychiatry at the Union Theological Seminary in New York, and a supervising analyst and faculty member of the C. G. Jung Institute in New York City. While her books cover a lot of different territory, this one, the book that speaks of how poison ivy can affect and change your life, is a most personal and intimate revealing of what analysis can really mean. Ulanov works in New York and summers in Connecticut, when she isn't traveling to present a workshop or lecture.